Weight Management

An American Yoga Association
Wellness Guide

Weight Management

An American Yoga Association Wellness Guide

The Powerful Program to Change the Way You Look and Feel Forever

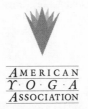

AMERICAN
Y·O·G·A
ASSOCIATION

Alice Christensen

The American Yoga Association

TWIN STREAMS
KENSINGTON PUBLISHING CORP.
http://www.kensingtonbooks.com

TWIN STREAMS BOOKS are published by

Kensington Publishing Corp.
850 Third Avenue
New York, NY 10022

ISBN 1-57566-636-7

Kensington and the K logo Reg. U.S. Pat. & TM Off.
Twin Streams and the TS logo are trademarks of Kensington Publishing Corp.

First Twin Streams Paperback Printing: January 2001
10 9 8 7 6 5 4 3 2 1

Printed in the United States of America

Photographs by Evelyn England, SAGE Productions
Hair and makeup by Estee Navarro and Ashley Kingston
Models: Pattie Cerar, Kent England, Linda Gajevski, Steve Honeyager, Steven Sanchez, Rodney Thompson
Book design by Melody Oakes

READERS PLEASE NOTE: *The techniques and suggestions presented in this book are not intended to substitute for proper medical advice. Consult your physician before beginning any new exercise program. The American Yoga Association assumes no responsibility for injuries suffered while practicing these techniques. The American Yoga Association does not recommend Yoga exercise for pregnant or nursing women or for children under 16 years of age. If you are elderly or have any chronic or recurring conditions such as high blood pressure, neck or back pain, arthritis, heart disease, and so on, seek your physician's advice before practicing.*

Acknowledgments

The author wishes to thank the staff, students, and friends of the American Yoga Association for their help with this book, particularly Pattie Cerar for general research assistance, Linda Gajevski for development and production, Stephen Grant for nutritional research and writing, and Patricia Rockwood for editorial assistance.

Table of Contents

Preface

When I began thinking about the title of this book, Weight Management, an image leapt into my mind of the difficulty of trying to stuff a large, unwilling, rebellious mass into a small rigid container fitted with a heavy door. If the door ever opens, the rebellious mass floods out in a fervor of freedom and takes back all the territory it had temporarily lost! It reminds me of the territory disputes constantly going on around the world, where a position hard won has to be constantly defended.

I have observed that those of us who have a tendency to maintain extra pounds on our bodies look upon a program of diet and exercise as a battlefield; one where, usually, battles have been fought many times and lost. It takes courage to face another battle, to lose and regain territory over and over again; in most of us, it strikes a chord of fear, a great inward fear of loss.

We rarely learn to respect the great depth of this fear. Having to lose a few pounds doesn't seem to be the end of the world, does it? In fact, weight counselors usually encourage participants by offering such statements as, "Try it, you'll like it. You will be proud of yourself." Such friendly, tranquilizing statements are meant to try to calm the inner hysteria of the body as it faces change and loss.

Long years ago, my great teacher Rama told me, "Yoga makes the rough road smooth." This simple statement made a tremendous impression on me then, and it is a part of my constant remembrance today. I have learned that by applying the ethics and standards of the practice of Yoga in all the victories and defeats of my everyday life, I can achieve balance within myself, and everything becomes possible.

I hope this book will help you to find a new way to approach your relationship with your body. The Yoga program presented in this book will help you see your goal of weight management less as a violent battlefield of constant struggle, and more as a process of learning how to create balance and confidence within yourself so that you can be what you want to be, and look the way you want to look.

Alice Christensen

Introduction

Weight management, which has traditionally been viewed as a personal problem, is now recognized as a serious national problem. Every year it seems that a greater percentage of the United States population is overweight to the extent that health is threatened. Extreme underweight, though perhaps not as widespread, is also a serious health concern of increasing proportions. The program outlined in this book will be most successful for those of you who are either mildly overweight or who are of normal weight and want to keep from gaining weight as you get older. If you are moderately to extremely over- or underweight, I strongly suggest that you seek professional help from a medical weight loss clinic or your personal physician, and use this book as added support for the changes you wish to make in your body.

Weight imbalance of any kind is often a signal of disease, especially if it occurs suddenly. Learning to manage your weight can help you to prevent illness, and it can help you with self-confidence and well-being. It is now known that people whose weight cycles up and down are at especially great risk for disease later in life. A greater percentage of our population is now older than ever before, and the trend is predicted to continue for the next few decades. Managing weight can increase confidence, fight illness, and help you maintain independence in the later years, when health often becomes more fragile.

Maybe this time ...

The main problem in weight management is that very few people are able to stay with a program for any length of time. January always produces a flutter of well-meaning attempts to restart diet and exercise routines to face the new year. We always hope that, maybe this time, the effect of our past indulgences can be totally repaired by the strong disciplinary action we are committing to now. We approach ourselves as a stern taskmaster, demanding immediate and perfect behavioral change. Since current statistics show that about 55% of adult Americans are overweight, I can easily picture at least half of America down on their knees on New Year's Day, promising that a new day is dawning on the eating front, envisioning a brand-new, slimmed-down body for the new year.

As the saying goes, the road to hell is paved with good intentions. How many of us try every new diet program on the market and fail each time? The only thing that grows thinner is our pocketbooks — and our confidence in ourselves.

The problem is not that we have not yet found the one true diet program that will work for us. The problem is that we are unable to keep our promise to maintain change in ourselves unless the whole person of us agrees. Exercise and nutrition are two important factors of a weight management program; a third component is the emotional factor. Successful change in the physical body depends upon the inner emotional body, and this kind of change is never possible without a balance between the two parts.

Your Two Bodies

This idea, that human beings have two bodies — the outer visible physical body that has a form, and the inner emotional/ spiritual body that is formless — is central to all Yoga philosophy. The practice of Yoga is the process of bringing the two bodies together in balance. In other words, you develop a harmonious relationship with yourself.

Play a game with me. Stand in front of a mirror and look quietly at your whole reflection. Imagine your body as the outward picture of your personality. Does it really display the real you — the "you" that you wish to use as your vehicle in this world? I am willing to bet that you will find fault with your reflection, thinking such thoughts as, "I may look like this, but actually I am really something else — something inside me that doesn't show on the outside." This split usually causes the inner being, the unseen side of you, to take the outer, physical side of yourself to task.

Yoga philosophy describes this as "an awareness of separateness." This then becomes the central focus of our physical being, when we try to find balance, compassion, and oneness with both our bodies: the spiritual inner body and the outer physical body. Yoga techniques help to transform the battlefield between the two parts of ourselves into a peaceful ground of understanding and appreciation of the needs of both of the bodies that make up our whole existence.

Stress and unhappiness are common occurrences when one or the other of the two bodies decides to go it alone. When the physical decides to suppress all emotional input from the spiritual body, for example, you will see a ruthless pattern emerging as denial and pain become the schedule for the day. This effect is markedly noticeable in the faces of people, especially athletes and many women, who suffer during bouts of extreme dieting. Both men and women who take a ruthless, demanding approach to the body without giving equal consideration to the inner unseen spiritual/emotional body take on a hard and dried-out appearance. The glowing softness of the body is gone — and so are most of the meaningful relationships in their lives.

Most weight loss programs deal mainly with the physical body, although a few placating statements may be thrown like a bone to the inner body, such as "You did it! You lost a pound!" or "This is not as terrible as you thought it would be." Such statements imply that the inner body's force can be harnessed to the wants of the outer physical body's desires for change; it is supposed to "buckle down" and behave, and that's that!

But this is not what happens. The inner emotional/spiritual body simply laughs and plays with us like an elephant with a mouse. It lets us have our game, and for a while the outer physical part of ourselves seems to control the show. We decide "I am going to change this body," and we go at it without the cooperation of both bodies in a friendly, productive bargain, one in which both sides feel that they win.

If this meeting does not take place, all efforts are bound to fail. The diet and exercise go on for a little while, but after some time the inner body tires of the game and comes back full force to return the outer physical body to its previous state, exactly as it was, very much like a fussy housewife who, every time someone moves a piece of furniture, hastily returns it to exactly the right position for her personal satisfaction.

Calling a Board Meeting with Yourself

Successful weight management can only take place happily when the two bodies are brought together. If you really want to change the way you look and feel once and for all, you must call a board meeting with yourself where both bodies are in attendance. Both bodies must be consulted for a happy agreement to the change.

It may be a difficult meeting at first, because the two bodies are not used to talking with each other, and this is not a meeting of equals! In fact, one has to wonder how the physical body ever got to the table at all. The emotional body is where your true strength lies; it sits like a big cat disdainfully observing a nervous squirrel or a rabbit. The physical body has no idea of the power of the emotional body; it marches in demanding change as if it had all the answers. The emotional/spiritual body listens and observes the physical's whining demands with lofty detachment. Each side maintains its separateness while the meeting goes on, and so nothing comes to agreement.

Try to imagine this scene played over and over again a hundred times as we try to change our lives. How many times have you tried to force your physical self to do something and failed? When the demands of the physical are put first, the body always suffers. I have observed people doing terrible things to their bodies in order to force a result. The body usually resents it so much that after a while it demands drugs, alcohol, or other distracting escapes to help ease the pain and upset.

Yoga philosophy believes that complete power lies in the inner body, the emotional/spiritual body, which never changes or dies. The fragile physical body, which is born and dies, actually only functions because of the strength and compassion of this inner body. If the two bodies can be encouraged to work together, the balance that is achieved makes any change possible.

This is the great contribution of Yoga techniques to those who practice it. The whole system of Yoga was designed exactly for this purpose. The word "Yoga" means "to join" or "to bridge." Yoga is a tool used to bring both parts of yourself together to work in harmony. When this happens, the constant inner battles with yourself transform into clear bright insights of intuition and practicality. The inner body then expresses its presence and power in all the activities of your life.

Yoga practice shows you how to make the board meeting between your two bodies a success. If you give the unseen inner body expression, it will stop all resistance. All it wants is expression, and that can be done happily only if the outer physical body welcomes it. This friendly attitude developing in yourself allows the strength of both bodies to come together in force, supporting all you want to do.

This book can teach you how to find balance within yourself so that fear of loss felt in both parts of yourself can be replaced with constant comforting support and feeding while change is taking place — very much the way a child is raised to maturity when conditions are the most ideal.

Working with Your Inner Body

American marketing tries hard to imply that there is "something more" than the advertised product that is displayed in the beautiful advertising that we see every day. However, it is difficult to portray the unseen. The outer physical body usually gets all the attention, while the inner spiritual side of ourselves lies beached and silent, erupting with force when it does not agree with the demands of the physical. The physical body says, "Now we are going to kiss this weight goodbye and be a new person!" — but what is the emotional reaction?

"Oh no!," the inner body says. "Wait a minute. I like things the way they are!" And the battle begins.

What a predicament! Yoga offers a way out by replacing all loss to both parties. Both will feel satisfied and be able to work happily together. Achieving this would mean that you become happy with the way you are. Those fortunate individuals who are happy with the way they are look beautiful. They shine with beauty from within that permeates their existence in the world. True, the exact perfection of the face and figure is usually not evident. It is never missed, however, because the beauty of the whole person displays itself, and we are enchanted.

Overview of This Book

I would like this book to give you a new way to approach weight management, whether you are trying to lose a few pounds or simply trying to maintain a normal weight. In this Introduction, I have tried to explain how Yoga can best help you change your outlook about weight management and increase your chances of success.

Sometimes it helps to educate yourself about the situation you are facing. In Chapter 1, I have outlined some basic information about overweight, including the most current ways that the medical community defines overweight, and how to figure your own starting point using the Body Mass Index (BMI). Chapter 2 provides a full description of our Yoga program, including a detailed discussion of how the various components of the program — exercise, breathing techniques, meditation, fantasy, mindful activity, and attention to nutrition — work together to help you meet your goals.

The Yoga program for weight management begins in Chapter 3, with complete instructions for the Yoga exercises that I feel will be most helpful to you. Along with the exercise descriptions, I have included some additional material about the effects and benefits of each technique and some links to important nutritional advice. The Yoga program for weight management continues in Chapter 4, with complete instruction in breathing techniques; Chapter 5, which teaches you how to relax completely and to meditate; and Chapter 6, which introduces you to some fantasy techniques that will enhance your success. This chapter teaches one of my favorite techniques: the "I Love You" meditation technique. This is a wonderfully effective technique that many of my students have used with great success to help them feel better about themselves and the changes they are attempting to make.

In Chapter 7, I introduce a way to incorporate more vigorous walking, swimming, or stationary cycling into your Yoga routine while practicing a contemplation exercise. This is a new technique that I developed especially for this book, and I hope you enjoy it.

No book on weight management would be complete without a section on diet and nutrition. Chapter 8 shows you how to modify your attitudes and tastes so that you can enjoy a satisfying and healthy diet, with instructions on how to determine your daily calorie requirements, design a personal eating plan either to maintain weight or to lose 1-2 pounds per week, and use supplements wisely. This chapter also presents a few sample menus to get you started.

At the end of the book you will find a complete Resources section that provides lists of support groups and organizations devoted to weight management, helpful Internet sites, and a reading list. This section also briefly discusses how to choose a qualified Yoga teacher and presents a complete, annotated list of the American Yoga Association's other books and tapes on Yoga for further study.

I hope this book will supply the impetus for creating a lifestyle that will take you through the rest of your years happily and with great beauty.

Cautions and Hints

Consult Your Physician

I advise all my new students to consult their physician before beginning Yoga practice. Although the exercises and techniques in this book are meant for beginners, and are presented in a way that makes them easy to learn and reasonably safe to practice, it is a good idea to make sure that you have no underlying health problem that could cause complications. Your doctor can best tell you what movements you may need to avoid or modify in order to minimize your risk.

It is easy to modify the exercises in the routine if you are severely overweight or physically limited due to a chronic health condition. For instance, many standing exercises, such as the Standing Sun Pose, can also be done in a chair. If you have any questions about modifying the exercises in this book, please write to me at the address printed in the Resources section.

Set Realistic Goals

Do not strain to do more than your body can do happily; this would violate the important Yogic ethic of Nonviolence, and if your body is feeling pain, you won't enjoy your practices. If you try to do too much at first, it may soon feel overwhelming. I would like you to enjoy Yoga practice, not look upon it as pain or drudgery.

Very few people have the time or desire to do a full Yogic exercise program every day, and so I suggest starting with the warmups and at least three exercises of your choice as your daily routine. Add more exercises whenever you wish, and gradually you can work into a fuller routine.

I would like to stress that your total daily commitment to Yoga practice, including exercise, breathing, and meditation, should not take more than one hour; the ideal time for beginners is 20 to 30 minutes per day. Yoga seems very easy to do; however, it creates a powerful effect that is not always apparent when you are first starting out, and practicing for over an hour might cause upset to your nervous system. Many times, in talking to people

I meet all over the world, I am dismayed to hear them say, "We do three hours of meditation every day," or "We always start with an hour of breath exercises." When I hear statements such as these, I have to suspect that the instructor is incompetent, because this intensity of practice is very hard on the nervous system. If students can truly meditate 10 to 15 minutes, that puts them at the top of my class! It takes many years to slip into long meditation, and it can never be forced. I suggest that you keep your daily routine short and interesting.

When to Practice

It does not matter what time of day you practice Yoga, although many people prefer early morning because their mind is not yet whirling with the day's activities. Some students find that they prefer to practice in the evening, because it helps them unwind from the day. Whatever time of day you choose, the most important thing to remember is to practice a little every day. Even if you practice only three exercises, three Complete Breath techniques, and a few minutes of meditation, you will continue to build an underlying momentum of regular Yoga practice that will eventually make it as easy and natural to do as brushing your teeth every day. You will miss it if you don't do it, because you find that you are enjoying it.

To make your practice even more effective, I suggest that you shower or bathe before you start your practice and fantasize all stress of the day washed away as you begin your routine with a fresh outlook.

Clothing, Equipment, Environment

Wear loose, comfortable clothing for Yoga practice, appropriate for the season. Try to keep these clothes separate so you use them only for Yoga practice. Do not allow yourself to become chilled; practice Yoga in an environment at normal room temperature. I regard overheated, saunalike environments as dangerous. It's best to practice Yoga exercises barefoot, but be sure to put on a pair of socks before you lie down for meditation in order to keep your feet warm. Wrap your upper body in a shawl or sweater when you meditate, because your body temperature will drop, and chill can upset your meditation period.

You do not need any special equipment to practice Yoga other than a large towel, blanket, or mat that you keep separate for Yoga practice. Setting aside one or two small, firm cushions for the seated breathing exercises may make you more comfortable. Choose a place in your home that is quiet and free from drafts. If you have small children at home, try to fit your practice into the times when they are asleep or at school, so that your attention is not split from what you are doing. Turn your telephone ringer off so you won't be startled by the loud noise, and be sure that you will not be disturbed by pets.

Scheduling

Although the different parts of your Yoga routine — exercise, breathing, and meditation — will work best if done consecutively, sometimes your schedule or family obligations may not allow that much time all at once. In that case, you can split your routine: For instance, you could practice breathing and meditation in the morning and your exercise routine in the evening.

Just be sure to practice a little every day without fail. I must repeat, however, that results are most quickly shown when all three components are practiced together.

Food, Caffeine, Alcohol, Medication

Wait about two hours after eating a large meal so that you are not practicing Yoga exercises on a full stomach. However, a light snack or beverage before exercising will not cause problems. Try to avoid practicing immediately after ingesting caffeine, and never practice Yoga under the influence of alcohol or so-called "recreational" drugs. If you are taking any prescription medications that make you drowsy, wait until the effects have lessened before starting your Yoga routine.

Women's Issues

Women should not practice Yoga exercises during the heavy days of their menstrual cycle. This is because the pressure of Yoga exercises on the internal organs may disrupt the natural hormonal changes of the body. Use the extra time for meditation, or spend a little more time on your walking exercises (see Chapter 7).

Many women begin a diet and exercise program after childbirth to help them return to their normal weight. We do not recommend that you practice Yoga exercises while you are nursing your baby because the chemical changes in your body caused by the compression on internal organs may affect your child. However, we do suggest that you continue your Complete Breath and meditation practice every day, as well as the Walking Contemplation exercise outlined in Chapter 7.

Supplemental Instruction

Yoga is best practiced alone, and I have designed this book to be your personal Yoga teacher. If you decide that you would prefer to supplement the course of study in this book with support from a local Yoga class, you will find, in the Resources, a discussion of some qualities to look for in a good Yoga teacher and a few suggestions about where to start looking. Also see the Resources for our excellent videotape that leads you through a basic 30-minute routine that you can do every day at home.

I hope that you enjoy this program of Yoga for Weight Management. If you have any questions about what you are doing, please feel free to write to me at the address given in the Resources.

Chapter 1

Some Facts About Overweight

Obesity is increasing so rapidly in the United States that weight maintenance and reduction is becoming a high public health priority. Today, more than half of all adults in the United States are overweight or obese. Excess weight is a common, serious, and difficult-to-treat problem. Anyone who has tried to lose weight can agree that long-term success is rare, since the lost pounds seem to eventually find their way back home.

Being overweight hurts in many ways. Excess weight causes high blood pressure, heart disease, strokes, some cancers, and diabetes. Being overweight can also hurt your inner self: Depression, anxiety, and low self-esteem can result from unwanted weight gain. Often the methods used to lose the weight are violent as well. Strategies such as extremely low-calorie diets, appetite suppressants, fat-blocking drugs, and surgery (liposuction, stomach-stapling, etc.) all cause violence to yourself in one way or another.

As I mentioned in the Introduction, repeated unsuccessful dieting may also be harmful to your health. The latest research confirms that "yo-yo" dieting, where your weight continuously cycles up and down as you try to diet for a short time, eventually give up, and then gain the weight back, may be very harmful to your heart and other body systems. This makes it essential to find a way to achieve and maintain a normal weight in a healthy way that will satisfy your inner body and help you continue your new eating and activity habits indefinitely; in other words, to permanently change your lifestyle.

Medical research makes it quite clear that prevention of weight gain is vastly preferable to trying to lose it later. Nearly every magazine at the check-out counter in the supermarket screams with headlines promoting a "new" diet or exercise program that makes it sound easy ("Lose 14 Pounds in Two Weeks!" "Five Days to Thinner Thighs!"). Evidence from our own experience, however, backed by countless research studies, shows that although it may seem easy to lose a few pounds in the short term, it is much more difficult to maintain the weight loss over the long term — unless you change your lifestyle. If you can do that, then keeping a normal weight becomes second nature. In other words, healthy, permanent eating and activity habits result in healthy, permanent weight loss.

Am I Overweight?

The definition of overweight has to do with the accumulation of excess body fat as a percentage of total body weight. No good method for measuring this directly at home has yet been found. Skin calipers, complete submersion in a water tank, and electri-

Add It Up!

Simple arithmetic will show you that over the long term, steady weight loss results in huge weight loss. If you lose "only" one pound per week, that is 52 pounds in one year; double those results if you lose two pounds per week!

cal impedance devices all tend to be inaccurate and unreliable except in the hands of a highly trained technician. Even then, changes within the body itself can add a surprising amount of variability: food and liquid in the intestines, menstrual cycle, intestinal gas, and even the amount of air in the lungs can all affect body fat measurements. A newer method, dualenergy x-ray absorptiometry, is the most accurate so far, but its use is currently restricted primarily to research centers.

Until recently, most people determined their "ideal" weight by reference to charts produced by the Metropolitan Life Insurance Company. The problem with these charts is that they were based on death rates of life insurance policy holders, who tended to be above-average-income younger white males. This hardly reflects the American population as a whole, and these "ideal" weights tended to be too high for younger people and too low for older Americans.

The Body Mass Index (BMI)

A better method, now commonly used by professionals and which you can easily figure out yourself, is called the body mass index (BMI). The chief limitation of the BMI is that it is unable to distinguish between muscle and fat — not a problem for most of us, but something to keep in mind if you are an athlete or unusually well-muscled. This simple measure, based on weight and height, is the most widely used index. It correlates very well with body fat percentage and predicts future health outcomes quite accurately.

To calculate your BMI, find your height (in inches) on the left side of one of the charts below and then read across to find your current weight (in pounds). The number at the top of that column is your BMI. For instance, if you are five feet nine inches tall (69 inches), and you weigh 155 pounds, your BMI is 23, which falls in the category of normal weight as indicated in Chart 1. Someone with the same height, but who weighs 175, has a BMI of 26, which would be considered mildly overweight, as indicated in Chart 2.

A BMI of less than 25 is in the normal range (Chart 1). "Mild overweight" corresponds to a BMI in the range of 25.0 to 29.9 (Chart 2), "moderate" from 30.0 to 40.0 (Chart 3), and "severe" in excess of 40.0. If you fall into the "mildly overweight" category (25 to 29.9 BMI), you are similar to about 90% of the overweight population, and you can benefit greatly from a lifestyle change such as the program outlined in this book. Those in the moderate category (about 9%) need some medical supervision, and the severe group (1%) have a serious condition that definitely calls for medical supervision and may even require surgery.

Chart 1: Normal Weights

Ht. in Inches	19	20	21	22	23	24	BMI
58	91	95	100	105	110	115	
59	94	99	104	109	114	119	
60	97	102	107	112	118	123	
61	100	106	111	116	121	127	
62	104	109	115	120	125	131	
63	107	113	118	124	130	135	
64	110	116	122	128	134	140	
65	114	120	126	132	138	144	
66	117	124	130	136	142	148	
67	121	127	134	140	147	153	
68	125	131	138	144	151	158	
69	128	135	142	149	155	162	
70	132	139	146	153	160	167	
71	136	143	150	157	165	172	
72	140	147	155	162	169	177	
73	144	151	159	166	174	182	
74	148	155	163	171	179	187	
75	152	160	168	176	184	192	
76	156	164	172	180	189	197	

Chart 2: Mild Overweight

Ht. in Inches	25	26	27	28	29	BMI
58	119	124	129	134	138	
59	124	128	133	138	143	
60	128	133	138	143	148	
61	132	137	143	148	153	
62	136	142	147	153	158	
63	141	146	152	158	163	
64	145	151	157	163	169	
65	150	156	162	168	174	
66	155	161	167	173	179	
67	159	166	172	178	185	
68	164	171	177	184	190	
69	169	176	182	189	196	
70	174	181	188	195	202	
71	179	186	193	200	207	
72	184	191	199	206	213	
73	189	197	204	212	219	
74	194	202	210	218	225	
75	200	208	216	224	232	
76	205	213	221	230	238	

Chart 3: Moderate Overweight

Ht. in Inches	30	31	32	33	34	35	36	37	38	39	40	BMI
58	143	148	153	158	162	167	172	177	181	186	191	
59	148	153	158	163	168	173	178	183	188	193	198	
60	153	158	164	169	174	179	184	189	194	199	204	
61	158	164	169	174	180	185	190	195	201	206	211	
62	164	169	175	180	186	191	196	202	207	213	218	
63	169	175	180	186	192	197	203	208	214	220	225	
64	174	180	186	192	198	203	209	215	221	227	233	
65	180	186	192	198	204	210	216	222	228	234	240	
66	185	192	198	204	210	216	223	229	235	241	247	
67	191	198	204	210	217	223	229	236	242	248	255	
68	197	203	210	217	223	230	236	243	249	256	263	
69	203	209	216	223	230	237	243	250	257	264	270	
70	209	216	223	230	236	243	250	257	264	271	278	
71	215	222	229	236	243	250	258	265	272	279	286	
72	221	228	235	243	250	258	265	272	280	287	294	
73	227	234	242	250	257	265	272	280	287	295	303	
74	233	241	249	256	264	272	280	288	295	303	311	
75	240	247	255	263	271	279	287	295	303	311	319	
76	246	254	262	271	279	287	295	303	312	320	328	

This book is primarily intended for the mildly overweight. If you have a BMI greater than 30, please consult your doctor first, and use this book to support and supplement your medical treatment.

Health Risks of Being Overweight

Being overweight is strongly associated with high blood pressure, high blood cholesterol, and reduced glucose tolerance; all of these conditions are in turn strongly associated with coronary heart disease (CHD). Overweight is itself an independent cause of approximately one-half of all CHD. The overweight have almost a three times higher prevalence of high blood pressure, and, in just the younger age range, a five times greater prevalence. In a study involving 115,000 nurses, those with BMIs of 29 or greater were over three times more likely to develop CHD than those in the lean category (BMI less than 21). Since more than 25% of American women between the ages of 35 and 64 have a BMI greater than 29, it is all the more important to reduce the prevalence of overweight.

Overweight is the single factor most strongly associated with Type 2 (non-insulin-dependent) diabetes, which has been estimated to affect more than 9 million Americans. Some studies indicate that as many as 90% of Type 2 diabetics are overweight. The risk of developing this form of diabetes increases from double, for mild obesity, to fivefold for moderate obesity, to tenfold for severe obesity.

The link between obesity and cancer is not as sharp, as the noted increase of risk begins with the moderately overweight —

those with a BMI in the lower 30s. For men, colon and rectal cancer increases with weight, and for women, the increases are seen in gallbladder, breast, cervical, endometrial, uterine, and ovarian cancers.

Several earlier studies clearly demonstrated that weight gain is also associated with a shortened life expectancy. Mortality rates from all causes for the heaviest people reach as high as 90% greater than for those of average weight. In a large study by the American Cancer Society, it was determined that those who were of average weight or who were from 10% to 19% below average had the lowest mortality rates.

Psychological Factors

A frequent misconception is that obese people overeat due to psychological disturbances: negative emotions such as inferiority, insecurity, sexual inadequacy, and so on. However, no study has ever been able to show a significant difference in the levels of psychological disturbance between the overweight and the general population. However, it is clear that being overweight often causes people to hate themselves and their bodies, and often it is this pain that eventually leads people to seek help for their weight condition. Most overweight people experience frustration and failure after repeated attempts to diet, and they are left with bitterness and contempt for themselves and an overall feeling of inadequacy. A sense of powerlessness and loss of control increases feelings of helplessness.

There seems to be a big difference, however, in individual emotional responses to being overweight depending upon one's race and socioeconomic status. Studies have shown that obesity is more common among those in a low socioeconomic group than in the American population as a whole. Among African-Americans and some Hispanic groups, there is greater acceptance of heavier body types. For many in these groups, being overweight may not feel very distressing. Since the emotional pain of being overweight, rather than health concerns, is what usually motivates overweight people to seek help, people who do not feel distressed about their weight are less likely to seek help in losing it. Though there is a lot to be said for accepting yourself no matter what your shape, the physical health consequences of being overweight are just as great among those who are more accepting of their shape as among those who feel distressed about their weight.

No matter what your heritage, the best approach from the point of view of Yoga is to observe your feelings and attitudes about overweight, especially those that may be violent toward yourself, and take the necessary steps toward losing weight.

Are the Health Risks Reversible?

Studies demonstrate that successful weight reduction can reverse the decrease in life expectancy associated with overweight. In fact, for one group of the population, obese individuals who successfully lost weight had mortality ratios comparable to persons who had never been overweight. Losing weight in itself is associated with lower blood pressure and cholesterol, and there is a reduced risk of coronary heart disease with weight loss of 10% or more. For those with high blood pressure, weight loss is preferred over medication to reduce blood pressure, because it lowers blood pressure further and results in a much healthier heart. For the diabetic, even modest reductions in weight resulted in improved blood sugar control and also lower blood fat and cholesterol levels. It is not necessary to achieve the ideal weight for significant benefits. Emotionally, those who lose weight generally experience dramatic improvements in mood, self-esteem, body-image, and social functioning.

Who's Dieting Now?

At any time, approximately 50% of American women and 25% of American men are dieting to lose weight.

Those who diet and fail — that is, those who lose significant weight and then quickly regain it — are possibly at higher risk for chronic diseases and shortened life. As I mentioned previously, such weight cycling may actually pose a greater risk to an individual's health than simply maintaining a constant weight. People with frequent or large fluctuations in body weight have a significantly higher risk of coronary heart disease and death. Everyone needs to be aware of the seriousness of both the hazards of being overweight and the hazards of exposing your body to a cycle of loss and gain. What matters most is gearing for long-term success so that you can successfully maintain weight loss.

Predispositions for Overweight

Genetics

There is a definite genetic predisposition to store excess calories as body fat, but the degree to which this contributes to overweight is not as clear. Studies of adoptees and twins suggest that genes are more important than the environment in the development of overweight. Studies of other types of relatedness indicate that there is perhaps a 25% genetic effect for overall body fat.

Metabolic Rate and Efficiency

Energy is measured in calories, and how your body uses energy is a simple ratio of calories in to calories out. You eat food (calories in) in order to supply your body with the energy to function (calories out). Even when you are at rest, your body is burning calories to breathe, to build and repair tissue, and to digest food.

The number of calories that your body uses to simply maintain itself while at rest is known as your metabolic rate. This rate is partly genetic, and so it is different for every person. Women generally have a lower metabolic rate than men, and for both sexes, metabolic rate declines with age. This is why most people gradually gain weight as they get older. As metabolic rate declines, your body needs fewer calories to do the same work; therefore, you need to either reduce your calorie intake or increase your activity level in order to maintain a constant weight.

If metabolic *rate* is how your body uses calories while you are at rest, metabolic *efficiency* is how your body uses calories while you are moving. This also varies widely among individuals and explains the exasperating fact that no two people obtain the same results from the same diet. If two people walk a mile together, one of them may need to burn 200 calories during that mile, while the other may need to burn only 100 calories. The person who burns the smaller number of calories has a more efficient metabolism. While we usually think of "efficiency" as a good thing, in weight loss terms it means that your body needs fewer calories in order to do the same work. So if you have a more efficient metabolism, in order to lose weight you have to eat fewer calories than someone whose metabolism is less efficient.

This is one reason that losing weight can often be frustrating; the more you lose, the greater your metabolic efficiency, and the less food it takes to keep the weight off! Many of us believe, deep down, that once we achieve our goal weight, we can go back to eating the way we did before, but of course the opposite is true, which is why in our program we stress changing your eating habits permanently. To make matters worse, if the frustration and sense of failure discourage you so much that you give up and resume eating the number of calories you were consuming before you started dieting (which was low enough to maintain a stable weight), that is now enough to cause rapid weight gain, quickly undoing several months of effort!

The "saving grace" in the weight loss process is increasing muscle mass through regular exercise. By moving the emphasis from simple weight loss to a comprehensive lifestyle change, the weight management program taught in this book counters the popular tendency to become "skinny-fat": losing weight without increasing muscle mass. The skinny-fat person will have a very low metabolism, so it is almost inevitable that the person will regain the weight that was lost. A fat body doesn't burn calories well, no matter what size it is! You have to convert fat to muscle. As you will see in the next section, muscle burns calories much more efficiently than fat, and the way to increase muscle mass is through exercise.

Physical Activity

A low level of physical activity probably plays a significant role in gaining weight, because the second component of our total daily calorie expenditure is exercise: all muscle contraction burns energy. Studies have shown that there is no difference between overweight and normal-weight people in the calories expended during exercise, but simply that the overweight are less active. Increasing physical activity can alleviate at least some of the decline in the metabolic rate that prolonged dieting can cause.

Fat Cells

Each person's tissues contain a various number and size of fat cells where the body stores excess fat, increasing cell size. The number of fat cells the adult body carries is primarily determined during infancy and adolescence, and most adults have a normal number of cells which grow in size as body fat increases. Those with the largest number of fat cells have the most difficult time losing weight; their losses tend to flatten out when their greater number of cells reach average size, and they are still overweight because of the greater number of fat cells.

It's as if your body has a built-in sensor that sends an alarm to your brain ("starvation imminent!") when fat cell size is reduced through dieting, causing you to eat more and your body to store more than usual as fat. No wonder weight loss can be difficult! This mechanism seems closely related to the degree of overweight; those who are severely overweight have a stronger alarm signal to eat more and store fat faster than those who are less overweight.

Set-Point Theory

Yet another factor in weight loss is that the body appears to recognize just one weight which it "defends" against efforts to raise or lower it. In other words, when faced with more calories than needed, the body compensates by becoming less efficient and using more calories than it really needs. When calories are short, during dieting for instance, the body compensates by becoming more efficient and increasing hunger. The body actually resists change, even though the weight may be judged too high or even too low for good health. The initial set-point may be high due to a genetically low metabolic rate.

If you have a normal weight set-point, it can be raised by eating excessive amounts of high-fat and high-calorie foods, and your body will then defend the new higher weight. If you succeed in losing weight steadily for several months or more (one or two pounds per week continuously), your body may be free of the regulation by set-point. However, if your dieting effort remains constant, but weight loss slows to a plateau, perhaps even starting to inch upward, then there is a good possibility that your body is resisting the change in weight by adapting to the reduced food intake. Successful weight reduction for this group will require a lifelong commitment to a lower calorie intake and increased physical activity compared with an average person of similar weight.

Chronic Dieting

As silly as it sounds, research has shown a connection between a history of dieting and overweight. Many people are driven to bingeing after time spent on a low-calorie diet. This is probably also a factor for those who try to lose weight by restricting food choices as well as those who try to reduce carbohydrates to extremely low levels. Binge eating may occur after or even during the dieting period. As I mentioned previously, the body often responds to low-calorie restrictions by reducing the metabolic rate. For some people, the reduction is far more than the actual reduction in weight. This increased metabolic efficiency makes additional weight loss more difficult to achieve.

The Fat-Carbohydrate Connection

Overweight people do not necessarily consume a greater number of daily calories than lean people. The difference is in the type of calories and what the body does with each type. Studies show that overweight people typically consume more fatty calories than leaner people, even though the total calories are similar. Some researchers even go a step further, claiming that high-fat foods in and of themselves cause higher weight gain than does the consumption of equally caloric high-carbohydrate foods.

Lean people, on the other hand, derive more of their calories from carbohydrates. Fatty calories are more readily stored in our fat cells; in fact, it is seven times easier for the body to store dietary fats as body fat than to convert excess carbohydrates to body fat! A high-carbohydrate, low-fat diet such as that outlined in Chapter 8, therefore, results in fewer calories being stored as body fat and more calories being used for fuel. This means that you have more energy for your Yoga routine, exercise, and daily activities.

Retraining Your Taste Buds

Our preferences obviously play a large part in what we eat. Overweight people tend to prefer high-fat foods more than lean people do. There is good evidence, however, that you can retrain your preferences, in effect resetting your taste buds' fat thermostat, by sharply reducing the fat in your diet. After several weeks of fat restriction, many people experience a greatly reduced craving for fatty foods. See Chapter 8 for some suggestions on how to retrain your taste buds.

Dangers of Low-calorie Diets

Low-calorie diets — 800 to 1,200 calories per day — do not meet the body's need for even resting calories. Do not try this at home! Before starting a diet this restricted, you need a physician's approval because of the metabolic effects of these diets as well as their ability to reduce body fat. There are many popular diet books with regimes in this range; they are often deficient in food variety, inadequate in nutritional quality, and often based on unsupported claims regarding such things as immune system, food combinations, or varying calorie intake to prevent reduction in the metabolic rate.

If you are contemplating a very-low-calorie diet, you should keep in mind that this level of restriction has negative metabolic effects, needs a physician's approval, requires vitamin and mineral supplementation, is extremely difficult to adhere to, and all too often simply leads to a cycle of severe dieting followed by bingeing. As I discussed previously, both severe dieting and bingeing are associated with overweight, and weight cycling is associated with heart disease and shortened life span.

Think long-term! Change your life! The maximum weight loss rate recommended is two pounds per week, achieved by any combination of increased activity and calorie reduction that burns about 1,000 more calories than are being consumed each day.

Characteristics of Those Who Succeed

People who succeed in keeping the weight off do so by emphasizing exercise, a gradual change in the diet, and sometimes group or individual therapy, rather than through self-control alone. These characteristics strongly apply to the mildly overweight.

If you exercise as well as diet, you are much more likely to maintain your successful reduction. The benefits of exercise include decreased appetite, increased metabolic rate, increased muscle mass, better overall health, and a better emotional state. Lifestyle change and consistency of exercise effort are key factors. As with dieting, the key question is "How much exercise will I be doing next year?" as opposed to "How many miles did I run today?" Beware of short-term overenthusiasm and focus on additional, gradual steps of exercise that are truly sustainable. If you don't enjoy it, you probably won't keep it up.

Chapter 2

How Yoga Can Help with Weight Management

The weight management program presented in this book is designed to help you resist becoming overweight or to be a strong support for those of you who are already overweight and wish to reduce. Essentially, the program is the same for prevention of weight gain or for weight loss; the only difference is in the number of calories you will consume (see Chapter 8). Our program is all about a lifestyle change: You will think differently, move differently, relax, breathe, and of course eat differently. By adopting this new lifestyle, you will have a much greater chance of preventing weight gain or of surviving the sometimes difficult path to permanent, successful weight reduction.

A new lifestyle is required, because the only way to lose weight successfully is to make a slow, sustained effort over months or even years. Similarly, the only way to prevent weight gain is to eat sensibly and maintain physical activity in a steady commitment indefinitely. This kind of commitment changes your life! You will start to gauge your success according to the long term — "I wish to weigh less six months from now" — rather than the short term — "I need to lose five pounds by Saturday!" You'll realize that such short-term dreams are unrealistic, because those first few pounds are only water loss and probably will be quickly regained. The real measure of success is losing body fat, and this takes a concerted, sustained commitment from both your physical and emotional bodies. Our program shows you how to nourish both your bodies so that they work together as a team and help you build the inner strength to keep a commitment to a long-term weight management goal.

The weight management program in this book offers several Yoga techniques and guidelines as part of a comprehensive behavioral approach to weight management that will help you build a new image of yourself. Among these techniques are physical exercises, breathing techniques, meditation training, fantasy exercises, attention to diet, awareness of ethics, and a special contemplation exercise to practice while doing mild aerobic exercise. Here are a few of the ways these techniques work:

• **EXERCISE.** The Yogic school of exercises, called asans, was developed for the body to maintain balanced mental and physical health. Yoga asans apply pressure to the glandular system of the body. This helps the body to stay strong and totally balanced. This glandular pressure also promotes the release of the chemicals, called endorphins, that cause feelings of well-being in the brain. This aspect of Yoga practice can be very helpful in relieving depression, anxiety, and insomnia. Yoga asans help to improve strength, flexibility, vitality, posture, and muscle tone, which will help you look and feel better, the idea being that the road to health lies in your own body. Yoga exercise contributes to a preventive system that helps avoid many common health problems associated with overweight, especially those that increase with age.

• **BREATHING.** Yoga breathing techniques nourish your inner body by helping to reduce anxiety and depression and create calm, clear, and creative thinking. Breathing techniques are designed to cleanse the nervous system, making its full function available for body needs. Breathing exercises also develop a depth of sensitivity which is very helpful in dealing with your inner emotional spiritual body. The effects are especially noticeable when you spend some extra time trying to begin a new relationship with yourself.

Many people first come to Yoga in order to reduce their stress responses. This is a wonderful "side effect" of practicing Yoga that will help you learn how to cope with the inevitable anxieties of life, especially when you are undergoing the additional stress of trying to lose weight. Many times, our usual response to stress is to eat; you will learn how to retrain yourself so that you will feel the same comforting feelings by doing breathing or meditation as you will from eating something that is not going to help you. You can always count on the fact that a few minutes of the Complete Breath (see Chapter 4) will help you quiet the whirlwind of anxious thoughts that accompany stress and often lead to overeating.

• **MEDITATION.** Yoga meditation techniques increase self-awareness and augment the balanced, calming effects of exercises and breathing techniques. Meditation is practiced so that the physical body and all inner conversation are silenced for a short time. This allows the intuitive voice, which is the language of the inner emotional body, to speak. This then is the gateway for expression that the inner spiritual body seeks, and it provides comfort and guidance from within.

• **FANTASY.** Guided Yoga fantasy techniques enhance self-esteem and counter the often frustrating sense of failure that serious weight reduction efforts may foster. Through practice of these techniques, which you can use throughout the day during many activities of daily life, you will learn that your inner thoughts and feelings determine your image of yourself and how you behave in the world. Regular practice of these fantasy exercises will help you build and sustain a new image of yourself as you wish to be.

• **MODERATE-INTENSITY EXERCISE.** Exercise helps to burn calories, build muscle, and improve cardiovascular fitness; in our program, we teach you how to perform more vigorous exercise with a Yogic mind of centered attention; a quiet meditative focus on your inner self. The best all-around moderate-intensity exercise is walking; it can be done by almost anyone, and it can be done safely while centering your attention on one of the contemplation topics introduced in Chapter 7. Walking can be done outside in any safe environment, or inside on any suitable treadmill. Other forms of exercise that will work with this technique are swimming and riding a stationary bicycle. If you are an experienced exerciser, you can probably adapt this technique to any form of safe exercise that you enjoy, such as jogging on a treadmill.

• **DIET.** A walk-through diet design process shows you how to determine your own calorie requirements and how to put together a sensible eating plan that builds health, satisfies hunger and cravings, and also provides for consistent, sustainable weight loss of one to two pounds per week. An important component of this section is recommendations for changing your taste preferences in foods to emphasize healthier choices while not giving up enjoyment.

These are the basic components of our Yoga Weight Management Program. Before starting to teach you the routine itself, I'd like to discuss the role of ethics in Yoga practice and weight management, and introduce you to a wonderful motivational technique that has worked well for many of my students.

Ethics in Yoga

Many times, Yoga is misrepresented as a religious practice. Yoga is not a religion; it is a way to find yourself, a joining, a bridge to the unknown parts of yourself. The science of Yoga provides tools that can be used by people of any faith or background to enhance their lives. One of the most important principles in Yoga is the practice of ethics. Yoga philosophy teaches that ethics are the gateway to the inner self. In other words, you can only fully experience the participation of your emotional/spiritual body with the help of an awareness and practice of ethical behavior.

Yoga holds great reverence for life, and for this reason, the ethic of Nonviolence becomes its mainstay. This is especially important when trying to manage weight. I have observed that most cases of overweight are due to one or the other of our bodies, the spiritual or the physical, acting with vengeance on the other. Imagine yourself looking into a mirror and saying "I hate the way I look!" Imagine your physical body feeling fear and upset because of impending attack, and the spiritual body saying,

"Wait a minute here, this is my production and don't fool with it!" This is not a peaceful place to play. Our game becomes a reality when we then punish ourselves with food, alcohol, or drugs, whipping ourselves with violent practices that throw us out of harmony and balance. (A complete discussion of Yogic ethical behavior may be found in my book *Yoga of the Heart* — see Resources.)

New Habits

Successful weight management can hardly ever be achieved if you divide your effort into "diet" days and "eat anything" days. To be successful, you need to start eating foods now that you can also look forward to eating a year or two or more from now.

Regular daily practice of the Yoga program outlined above will prepare your physical body to join with your inner emotional body without pain or upset. The results show very quickly. You should feel the difference in just two or three days. It is hard to describe this change, because the body does not change quickly, but the feelings that accompany regular practice are so pleasant that you won't want to give it up. For this reason, those who take up the practice of Yoga rarely ever stop. Thousands of people who have bounced around from one weight management program to another, unable to maintain a daily discipline happily, now look forward to their daily practice of Yoga. You will never fear it; in fact, you will really miss your practices if you don't do them. You don't have to go to a class to achieve this effect; practicing at home alone with this book, or with a class videotape such as our "Basic Yoga" (see Resources), will give you wonderful results.

A regular daily routine of Yoga exercises, breathing, meditation, and fantasy, even if it lasts only a few minutes, will produce happy, comforting expression from the inner emotional body. When this happens, healing begins. The two bodies at your inner board meeting can finally talk to each other as the rift of separateness heals, giving you the full power to be what you want to be.

Why Do We Eat?

In its approach to diet and nutrition, Yoga takes the view that food functions in many more ways than as simple nourishment for the body. In talking with students over the years, and from my own personal experience, I find that people who tend to be overweight do not eat because they are hungry. Something unseen drives them to eat more — and more often — than they need to. Most of us have been trained to ignore our inner feelings and push on bravely in whatever is demanded of us. This habit will seriously upset the inner emotional body by blocking its expression. When this happens, the physical body panics and looks for help.

Many times that help lies in food, and the constant comforting needed by the individual puts on the extra bulk to provide protection from attack. The same thing happens in extreme starvation. People believe that if they eat, they will be attacked, and so they stop eating. Eating too much — or refusing to eat — becomes a response to many emotions, most often fear. Those who suffer extreme over- or underweight are always afraid of attack.

Fear becomes a serious detriment when you try to change, because it forces you to maintain a stationary position, holding on to all the habits that made you subject to fear in the first place.

Usually it doesn't matter what type of food it is; what matters is that something is in the mouth at the time the hidden feeling of fear comes forward. I believe that this habit comes from the inner body's fear of loss. Using Yoga techniques daily can comfort you and help you become aware of the fear response, so that you don't feel the urge to eat each time an upset occurs. The important key to this practice is noticing when you are feeling fear or upset in yourself, and then feeling the power to be able to do something about it. This increased awareness invites input from your inner emotional spiritual body. When this happens, the upset usually goes away and balance can be achieved.

The Wrist Tape Technique

This is a wonderful motivational tool that you can try to help you succeed in your weight management program. My students have great luck with this technique, which they use when they want to change something in their behavior. It is extremely successful in the practice of ethics or any other behavioral change that you wish to attempt. Let's say you wish to become aware of how often during the day you succeed in eating foods that will help build your new vision of yourself.

To try this exercise, simply place a small piece of nonirritating tape, such as first aid-type adhesive tape or painter's masking tape, on the inside of your wrist or on a watch band. Draw a line down the middle to make two columns: the left column for positive, and the right one for negative. Each time you eat or drink, make a mark in one of the two columns depending on how you feel about what you have done for yourself. This will show you how you are dealing with producing the vision in yourself that you want to become. At the end of the day, stick the tape on your refrigerator door. By the week's end you will see a row of tapes indicating how you have progressed in becoming aware of what is really happening in your daily diet practices.

Using a Wrist Tape to Practice Nonviolence

Here is what one student wrote to me about her practice of this technique: "When I caught myself in a violent thought and made a mark, it was as if I was able to let it go, instead of grinding and grinding about whatever it was that was upsetting me. I know this connection is nebulous, but somehow it helped me to see that nothing is outside of myself; that all those things that I thought were out there upsetting me were actually reflections of my own self — my unconscious self that I tend to forget to talk to, even though I've been trying every day to take time out to give it voice. It's made me take another look at the way I've been trying to run my life."

This practice promotes great respect for yourself because it shows you the great effort you are putting into your lifestyle change. When you are able to perceive the effort clearly, you will be able to really congratulate your inner emotional spiritual body for its support in the process. This will begin to bring you together with your emotional self in a nonviolent process that will develop a friendly support within yourself for what you want to do.

Be Kind to Yourself

Now you are ready to begin our complete Yoga Weight Management Routine. Don't worry if you cannot do the complete routine all at once. In fact, if you have not exercised in a long time, it will be much more beneficial to start slowly, doing one or two exercises each day and adding techniques as you gain strength and stamina. Always try to practice a little every day, however, and practice the exercises, breathing, and meditation together for best results. This daily consistency will give momentum to your efforts and result in quicker and longer lasting results.

Here is a suggested schedule for the first week, incorporating each of the five parts of our program, illustrating how to increase your practice gradually over several weeks:

Exercise

All warmups, plus three exercises (add 1-2 new exercises each week)

Breathing

3 Complete Breaths (add 3 repetitions each week until you reach one minute total; next try the Cooling Breath technique, starting with 3 repetitions and adding 3 each week until you reach one minute; next add the

Alternate Nostril Breath and build up to one minute; finally add the Soft Bellows Breath and build up to one minute. Your total practice of breath techniques at one sitting never needs to exceed four minutes. Of course, you can practice breathing techniques at other times of the day as described in Chapter 4).

Meditation

5 minutes (add 3 minutes per week until you reach 20 minutes — about six weeks; stay at this length of time indefinitely, or continue to 30 minutes in 3-minute intervals as before).

Fantasy

"Creating a Vision of Yourself." (Practice this every day for one week, then try a new fantasy exercise the same way during the following week and the week after. Then alternate techniques as you wish, or practice them combined with your activity program as described in Chapter 7).

Walking Contemplation

5-10 minutes per day (add 5 minutes per week).

Diet

In the first week, choose just one change to make in your diet; for example, switch from 2% milk to fat-free; or, instead of two cookies for dessert, eat one cookie and one apple. See Chapter 8 for more suggestions. In week two, make another small change in your diet, and determine your calorie count according to your goal weight; study the sample menus. In week three, make a third small change in your diet and follow one of the sample menus for one or two nonconsecutive days that week. In week four, add a day on your new calorie count. Starting in week five, follow the suggested calorie count for at least 6 days out of 7.

Some of my students enjoy recording their progress in a chart form. If you like, create a chart or a journal that records your goals for each of the six parts of the program for each week, and include a space to write in how you met your goals, what you experienced during your fantasy exercises or while meditating, and how you felt about yourself every day. Here is a sample:

Week 1
Exercise

Goal — *warmups and 3 exercises.*

Result — *did warmups only for 2 days, then added the Triangle poses and Standing Sun Pose. Felt a little stiff in the back of my legs, but it went away by the end of the week. Added the Cobra V-raise.*

Breathing

Goal — *3 Complete Breath exercises*

Result — *Loved this technique! Found myself doing it while waiting in the doctor's office Wednesday. Helped me feel less nervous.*

Meditation

Goal — *5 minutes*

Result — *Felt like I was just lying there thinking about my "to do" list. About the third day, felt myself stop talking to myself for a few seconds. By the end of the week, I fell asleep.*

Fantasy

Goal — *"Vision of Myself"*

Result — *Had trouble seeing anything but the things I don't like about myself at first. After a few days, had to admit I like my smile, and found myself smiling more into the mirror in the mornings.*

Walking

Goal — *5-10 minutes*

Result — *Got overenthusiastic the first day: walked around the neighborhood for about a half hour — sore the next day. Walked 5 minutes anyway. Felt better. Missed only one day this week.*

Diet

Goal — *make one small change in diet*

Result — *Decided to try milk in my coffee instead of cream. Succeeded every day except Sunday.*

Always maintain a constant, friendly approach with yourself, reminding yourself that this is a lifetime change that slowly and steadily will build solid supporting blocks of health, strength, and happiness for yourself and your new way of living.

Chapter 3

Yoga Exercise for Weight Management

In this chapter you will find a complete Yoga exercise routine especially designed to be helpful for weight management. The routine is organized so that the easiest exercises are presented first, so start at the beginning. If you have not exercised in a long time, I suggest that you begin by practicing only the warmups (pages 51-61) and then three additional exercises. Add two or three exercises each week until you are able to practice the full routine.

How to Practice Yoga Exercises for Best Results

Breathing

It may be tempting to plunge right in and just follow the pictures, but if you do you will miss the important instructions about how to breathe during the exercise. Breathing is a crucial element of Yoga exercises, and each pose or movement has a particular breathing pattern that contributes greatly to its effect. Read completely through the instructions before beginning, in order to be sure you are breathing correctly as well as to avoid injury.

Always breathe through your nose, both inhaling and exhaling. If you concentrate on the steamlike sound of your breath as you move through the routine, you will notice a wonderful silence in your mind that will naturally lead you into a very deep, restful meditation. (See Chapter 4, p. 100, for how to make the steamlike sound with your breath.)

The exercises have been laid out in a sequence from standing to seated to lying down. The transition between exercises is often where concentration is lost. Try to keep your attention on your breath throughout the entire routine, and try to stop all conversation inside your head.

Most exercises are movements matched with either an inhalation or an exhalation. You breathe in to a count of three, hold for a count of three, breathe out for a count of three, hold for a count of three, then rest for a count of three. This focuses and settles your mind on the proper position of body, breath, and mind. This does not have to be a slow count! Any time you feel winded, and especially when holding a pose, you can increase the speed of your three-count in order to avoid strain.

Work at Your Own Pace

Yoga exercises should not hurt. Be kind to your body! Move slowly and carefully, paying attention to how your body feels at all times. I can't stress enough how important it is to work at your own pace. As I mentioned previously, if you haven't exercised in a long time, don't try to do the entire routine all at once. In fact, it's probably a good idea to do only one repetition of each exercise the first few times you try it, just to make sure there is no movement that will aggravate a back condition or other physical problem you may not be aware of. When you are sure that there is no pain, do the exercise three times as instructed. As I've said previously in this book, the important thing is to practice at least three exercises every day. When you practice every day, your strength and endurance will gradually increase until you can do the entire routine.

If some of the exercises are too difficult, practice them at only half capacity until you become more proficient. Remember, Yoga is a nonviolent practice. If you haven't exercised in a while, you may experience some tightness in your joints and muscles, especially in the back of your legs when you practice forward-bending exercises. With daily practice, you will notice a big difference in your stretching and bending ability in just a few weeks.

Most exercises call for about three to five repetitions. If this is too much at first, just go at your own pace, remembering that Yoga works best in small steady increments.

Warmups

The first several exercises in your routine gradually introduce your body to the idea of exercising. They are simple stretches that work on the major muscle groups of the body, gently stretching the long muscles of the legs and back, gently bending the spine, increasing circulation, and loosening the joints of the shoulders, hips, and spine. Remember to breathe through your nose at all times and concentrate on the sound of the breath. Pay attention to how your body feels, and move only to the point before it starts to hurt; Yoga is a nonviolent practice. Eventually you will be able to do the whole movement. In the following routine, the warmups begin with the Shoulder Roll and end with the Lazy Stretch.

Stress is a pervasive force in our daily lives that can cause us to fear movement. This is especially so when we are afraid of attack, no matter what the source, or whether it's justified or not. It's as if the body feels such a need for protection that it carefully guards its movements so as not to be hurt further. The Shoulder Roll and other warmups will help your body to gradually feel more relaxed about the movements that lie ahead in the routine so that it doesn't feel so frightened.

The B-complex vitamins and vitamin C are very important for helping support your body in the management of stress responses. See Chapter 8 for more information about how to be sure your diet includes enough of these nutrients.

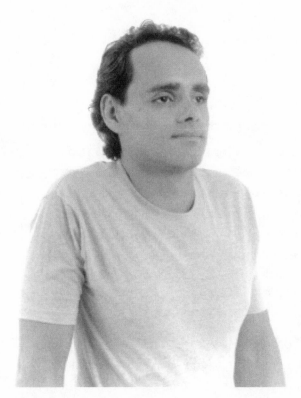

(1) Shoulder Roll

SHOULDER ROLL

Benefits: Loosens shoulder joints and upper back.

Breathe normally throughout this exercise, and always breathe through your nose. Stand with feet parallel and arms hanging loosely at your sides. Lift both shoulders up toward your ears (without bending your elbows) and rotate your shoulders in circles, first forward, then backward, at least 5 times in each direction (1). Keep your arms and hands hanging loosely.

Learning to relax at will is a vital skill for a Yoga student. Every exercise provides an opportunity to learn a different way to relax your body and mind. Sometimes the best relaxation comes after an exertion. In the Arm Circles, your heart and the rest of your respiratory and circulatory systems are energized, so your entire upper body feels flushed with life-giving blood that is packed with oxygen. Enhance the relaxed feeling by shaking out your arms and shoulders after this exercise.

Sometimes people who have trouble relaxing during the day also have trouble going to sleep at night or staying asleep. If this applies to you, try cutting out caffeinated beverages after 5 pm. Practice a few warmups just before bed, and practice two or three Complete Breaths when you lie down. Try to think of nothing except the sound of your breath. Then meditate yourself to sleep with the "I Love You" technique (see page 118).

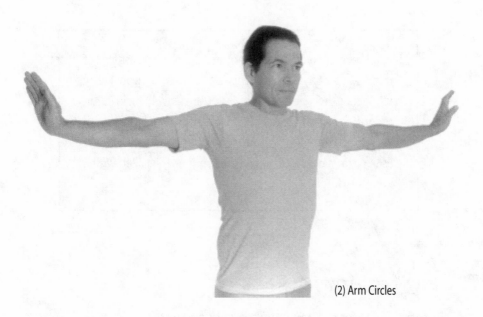

(2) Arm Circles

ARM CIRCLES

Benefits: Increases circulation; strengthens back and shoulders; improves range of motion of shoulders; limbers upper back, chest, and midback.

Stand with feet parallel. Lift your arms straight out to the sides, fingers flexed and palms facing outward (2). Maintaining this position, rotate your arms first in large, slow circles and then in small, faster circles, 5 to 8 times in each direction. Breathe normally throughout. Finish by shaking out arms and shoulders.

In this exercise you are concentrating on the movement of just one part of your body. This is a wonderful opportunity to practice the quiet feeling that you are striving for in meditation. Stop all inner conversation with yourself; such conversation dilutes the effect of the exercise. Instead, imagine as you turn your head slowly that your head is filled with a great silence.

NECK STRETCHES

Benefits: Releases tension in upper back and neck.

Cautions: If you have disk problems in your neck, check with your doctor before trying this exercise.

Breathe normally throughout this exercise. Start by gently bending your neck forward and slightly to the right, so your chin reaches down toward your collarbone. Place your left palm on your neck to monitor the stretch (3). Hold for several seconds, breathing normally. Repeat on the opposite side. Release, and gently turn your head from side to side.

If you have no neck problems, you may add a Head Rotation: Place your hands on your hips or let them hang straight down, and keep your shoulders relaxed. Gently bend your head to the left, bending your ear over your shoulder and being careful not to lift your shoulder (4). Roll your head forward, chin toward your chest, and continue rolling your head over toward the right shoulder, then back slightly, then over to the left to complete the circle. Repeat, slowly, twice more to the left and then 3 times to the right. Keep shoulders relaxed at all times; the only parts of your body that should move are your head and neck.

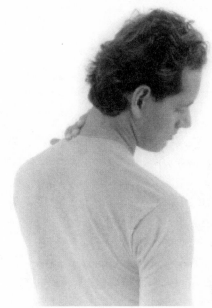

(3) Neck Stretches

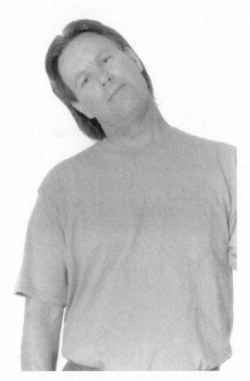

(4) Head Rotation

The previous warmups focused on your upper body. With the Elbow Twist exercise, you will begin to feel the effects of improved circulation in your entire body. Continue the mental exercise described for the Neck Stretches. Imagine yourself filled with a vast silence. Imagine the silence spreading throughout your entire body. You will feel a restful feeling of relief while you slowly twist from side to side. Your physical body will loosen up and begin to lose its fear of movement. Your emotional body will feel centered and focused.

ELBOW TWIST

Benefits: Limbers spine; improves respiration and posture.

Stand with feet a few inches apart, and be sure your back is straight. Raise your arms to chest height, bend your elbows, and place one hand on top of the other. Breathe in completely to a count of three while looking forward, then breathe out slowly to a count of three as you twist toward the left, leading with your left elbow. Look around to the left so your entire upper body is gently twisted (5). Hold for a count of three, then breathe in to a count of three as you return to face front. Repeat 3 times to each side, alternating.

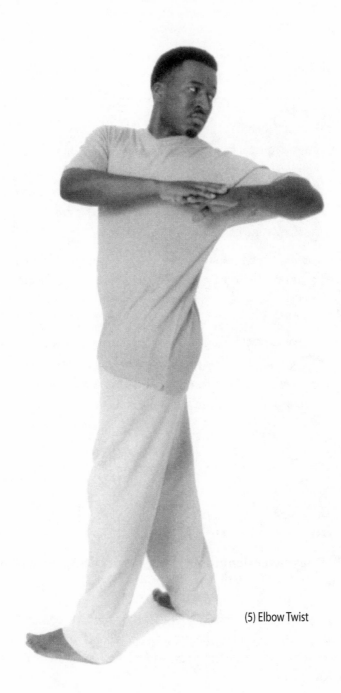

(5) Elbow Twist

My teacher Rama used to say that this simple exercise was the key to total body health. It uses all the major muscle groups, and affects the nervous, circulatory, glandular, and respiratory systems. Practicing this exercise will prevent the development of a swayback or hunchback. This exercise invites a mystical connection with the sun.

Nothing happens in the physical world without first happening in the mind. If you want to build a chair, for example, you first have to fantasize the chair in your mind; then you pick up the saw and hammer to build the chair. Similarly, when you practice Yoga exercises, you attain best results if you fantasize the changes you want to see in your body. As you practice the Full Bend, visualize your body stretching out until it becomes taut and lean and brave.

FULL BEND AND HOLD
(Paschimottanasan Prep.)

Benefits: Releases tension in upper back and neck; helps to reduce a large stomach.

Cautions: If you start to feel faint while bending forward, bend only halfway down, but still be sure to let your head, arms, and hands hang forward loosely when you breathe out. Hold on to a chair back or railing with one hand to protect from falling.

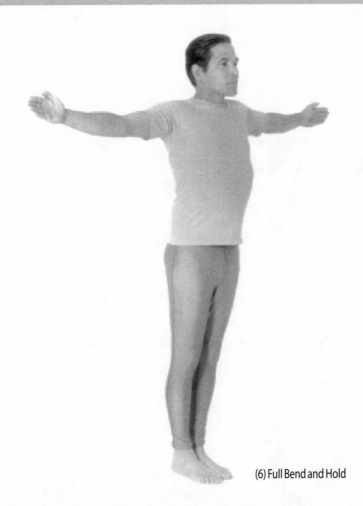

(6) Full Bend and Hold

Stand with feet parallel, a few inches apart. Breathe out completely. Breathe in to a count of three as you slowly raise your arms up and out to the sides, parallel to the floor (6). Stretch back a little as you hold your breath in for a count of three, then breathe out to a count of three as you slowly bend forward, leading with your hands, until you are as far forward as possible. Let your whole body go limp and hold your breath out for a count of three (7). Now breathe in to a count of three as you slowly come back up, bringing your arms out to the sides again. Continue to breathe in as you straighten up and breathe out as you bend forward, matching your breath to your movement. Repeat 3 to 5 times.

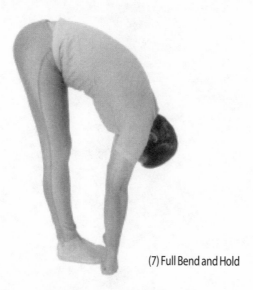

(7) Full Bend and Hold

After the last repetition, breathe out and come forward once again, but let your arms relax toward the floor and hold the position, breathing naturally. If you can reach the floor comfortably, let your fingers curl slightly. Just go limp and relax. Let your head hang so your neck stretches. Don't hold your breath. Hold for several seconds, then slowly stand up.

When my great teacher Lakshmanjoo was teaching me about the Yogic ethic of Tolerance, he said that a true hero is the person who can take one more step. Practicing Yoga techniques every day will build your endurance and courage so you can keep going no matter what happens. The Lazy Stretch exercise is particularly beneficial for improving lung capacity, balance, and stamina, giving your physical body the support it needs to remain strong.

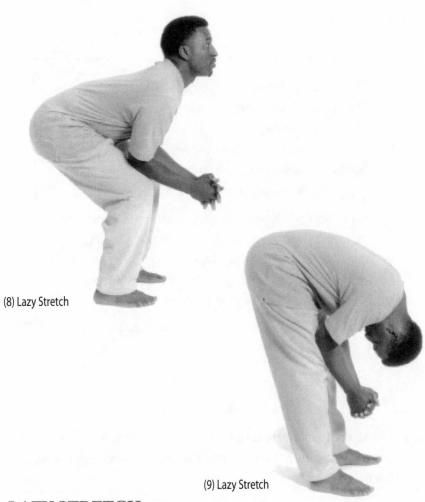

(8) Lazy Stretch

(9) Lazy Stretch

LAZY STRETCH

Benefits: Stretches back of legs and lower back; strengthens ankles and calves; improves respiration.

Stand with feet shoulder width apart. Bend your knees and rest your forearms on your knees with hands clasped. Breathe in to a count of three as you look up, arching your back slightly (8). Hold for a count of three. Breathe out to a count of three as you straighten your legs while keeping your forearms on your knees (9). Tuck your chin toward your chest. Hold for a count of three. Repeat 3-5 times.

The symbol of the triangle is central to Yogic philosophy. The upward-pointing triangle represents the unseen support of the universe, while the downward-pointing triangle represents the entire manifested world. When the two triangles are superimposed one on the other, it represents harmony and balance in the universe and within ourselves.

The Alternate Triangle helps you attain balance in body and mind while improving muscle tone, concentration, and endurance. When you turn and bend from side to side, you will feel the extra compression in your abdomen and the improved circulation to your hands and feet.

ALTERNATE TRIANGLE (Trikona Hasthasan)

Benefits: Stretches and strengthens muscles in the back, hips, and shoulders; compresses internal organs, stimulating metabolism; improves circulation to legs and feet.

Separate your legs as far apart as you can comfortably, and point your toes straight ahead. Breathe in to a count of three as you stretch your arms out to the sides (10), then breathe out to a count of three as you bend toward your left leg. Remember to keep your knees straight but not locked. Grasp your left ankle firmly with both hands, bend your elbows, and pull gently, keeping your knees straight and tucking your chin into your chest (11). Hold the position and your breath for a count of three. Breathe in to a count of three as you return to the starting position with arms outstretched. Repeat 3 times to each leg, alternating.

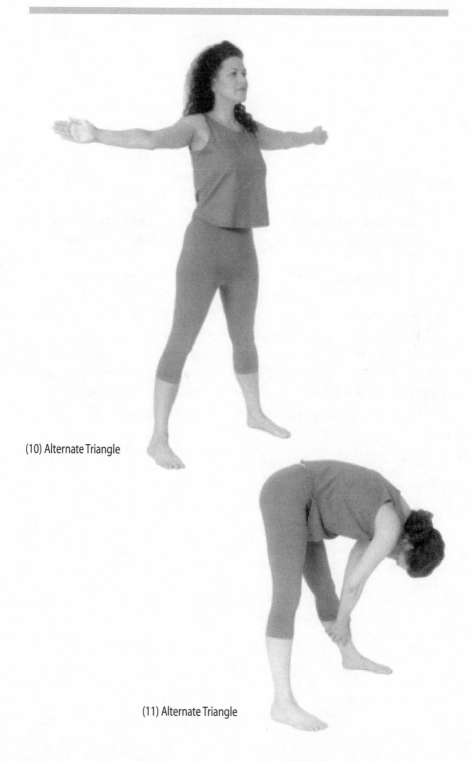

(10) Alternate Triangle

(11) Alternate Triangle

SIDE TRIANGLE (Uttihita Trikonasan)

Benefits: Limbers back, legs, hips; limbers intercostal (rib cage) muscles; improves respiration and balance; strengthens heart.

With feet still separated, toes pointed forward, breathe in completely to a count of three, arms outstretched as in photo 10, then breathe out to a count of three as you bend sideways toward the left, sliding your left hand down your left leg. Bring your right arm up and over your head, keeping it as straight as possible and parallel to the floor if you can; stretch from your waist (12). Look at a spot on the wall straight in front of you. Hold your breath out for a count of three. Breathe in to a count of three as you return to the starting position. Repeat 3 times to each side, alternating.

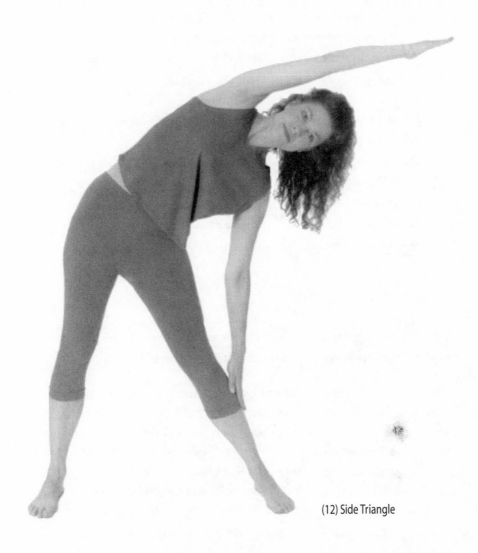

(12) Side Triangle

Self-confidence is one of your most important assets while you work on managing your weight, and one of the best ways to increase confidence is to visualize yourself the way you want to be. As the image solidifies in your mind, your body will begin to take that shape. The T Pose is especially helpful in improving balance and steadiness. You will see and feel a new gracefulness in your body if you practice this exercise regularly. Visualize yourself as you want to be and hold that picture in your mind as you hold the position.

T POSE (Virbhadrasan)

Benefits: Strengthens legs and back; improves vigor; tones abdominal organs; increases concentration, memory, and mental poise.

When you are first learning this position, stand three to four feet from a chair or other support. Lean forward and hold on to the support with both hands. Lift your left leg in back as high as you can (ideally, parallel to the floor). Alternatively, brace yourself with both hands on the knee of your supporting leg. Keep your right (supporting) leg straight. Your torso and left leg should be in a straight line parallel to the floor. Keep your neck straight, breathe naturally, and look at a spot on the floor (13).

When you feel steady, release your grip on the support and place your palms together, pushing your arms out parallel to the floor. Relax your breath and breathe naturally. Look forward at your hands (14). Lower your leg and return to a standing position. Rest. Repeat on the opposite side. (This exercise is only done once on each side.)

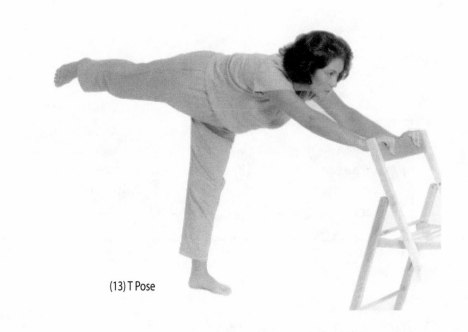

(13) T Pose

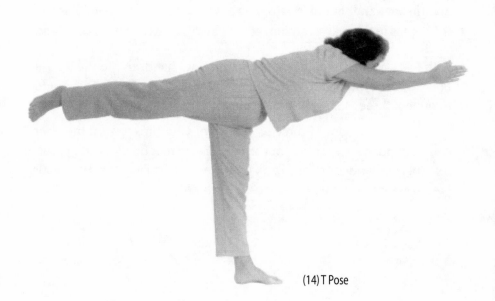

(14) T Pose

This exercise allows the heart to expand. I have found this exercise extremely helpful in correcting fertility problems. It may enhance sexual potency if practiced regularly and balanced with two or three other exercises of your choice.

COBRA V-RAISE (Svanasan)

Benefits: Strengthens legs, back, shoulders, and rib cage; improves bone mass in arms and shoulders; strengthens heart; improves functioning of the organs in the pelvic region; reduces body fat; stretches back of legs.

With feet parallel, bend forward and walk your hands out to the V position (15). Tuck your head, push your heels to the floor, and breathe out to a count of three. Hold your breath out for a count of three.

Breathe in to a count of three as you lower your hips toward the floor and arch your back, keeping your arms and legs straight, supporting yourself only on hands and feet. Look up toward the ceiling (16). Hold your breath in for a count of three. Repeat 3-5 times.

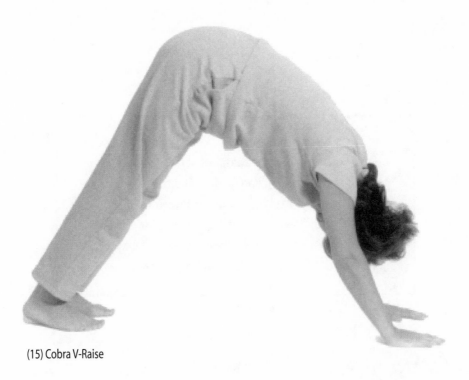

(15) Cobra V-Raise

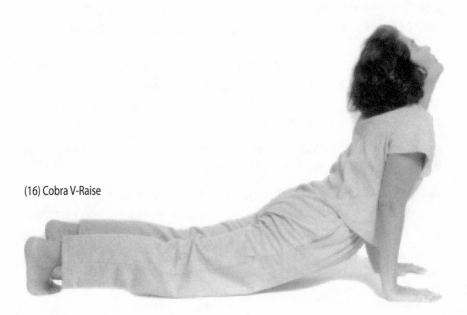

(16) Cobra V-Raise

There is a reason this exercise is called the "sun pose": it brings radiant, all-around health, just as the sun is the earth's source for nourishment and growth. The best way to practice this exercise is to visualize the sun as you raise your arms and breathe in deeply. Hold this image in your mind's eye as you complete the exercise, then rest. The radiant, life-giving properties of the sun will fill your heart and body.

STANDING SUN POSE (Padahasthasan)

Benefits: Improves functioning of digestive and circulatory systems; exercises heart and lungs; limbers and strengthens legs and back.

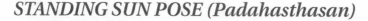

Stand with feet parallel. Keep your knees straight but not locked. Breathe out. Breathe in to a count of three as you raise your arms in a wide circle to the sides (17) and overhead. Stretch and look up at your hands (18). Hold your breath in for a count of three.

Breathe out to a count of three as you bend forward from the waist, keeping your hands together and your head between your arms (19).

Grasp your ankles or calves firmly, bend your elbows, tuck your chin, and pull your torso toward your legs (20). Be sure to pull by bending your elbows instead of straining your lower back. Keep your knees straight and hold your breath out for a count of three. [NOTE: If you have back or neck problems, bend only halfway down, and do not pull in with your arms.]

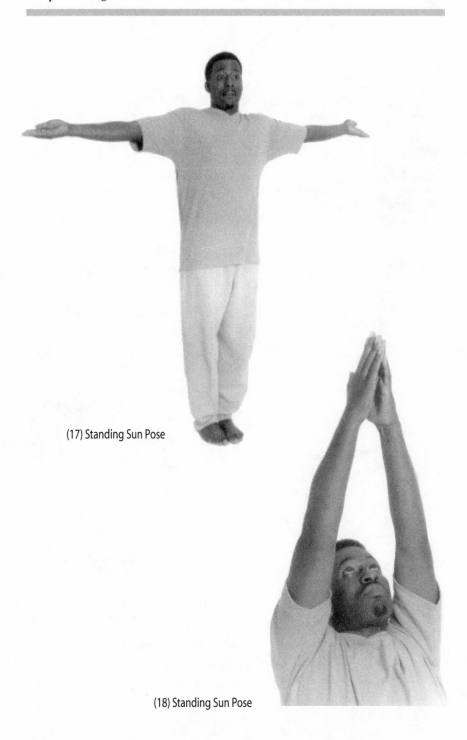

(17) Standing Sun Pose

(18) Standing Sun Pose

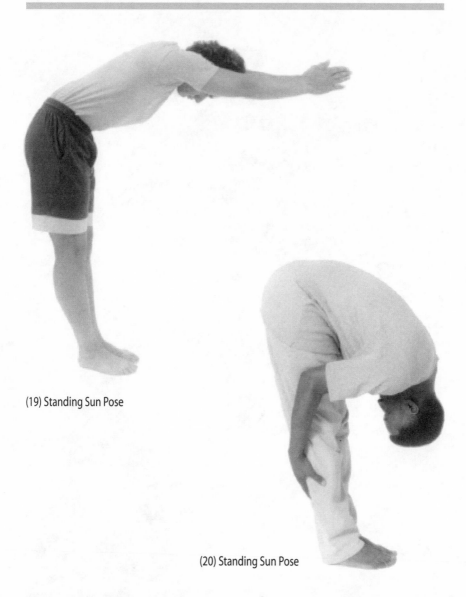

(19) Standing Sun Pose

(20) Standing Sun Pose

Release and breathe in to a count of three as you slowly straighten, bringing your arms in a wide circle to the sides and over your head again. Look up and stretch as in photo 18. Hold your breath in for a count of three. Breathe out to a count of three as you slowly lower your arms to your sides. Repeat 3 times.

In Yoga, the nervous system is often pictured figuratively as covered with a sort of slime or mucus that contributes to feelings of sluggishness, dullness, and imbalance. Exercises such as the Whirlwind create an internal heat that clears away this covering so the nervous system becomes bright and active. You will feel this heat in your body as you practice.

THE WHIRLWIND (Nauli)

Benefits: Compresses internal abdominal organs; strengthens abdominal muscles; stimulates digestion; reduces body fat; stimulates reproductive system. Many people feel a very pleasant warmth building up during the exercise.

Caution: If you have a lower back problem, begin this exercise seated on the edge of a chair (see note, p. 75), as there is greater strain on your back when standing.

Because this exercise requires you to hold your breath out for quite a while, it can be a bit strenuous until you learn it. Be sure to read through the entire set of instructions before beginning. An excellent warm-up exercise, which will strengthen your abdominal muscles, is the Easy Sit-up (page 87). Practice it for a few weeks until your strength increases. If you can easily do 15-20 sit-ups in a row, you should be able to perform the Rising Breath and Whirlwind exercises without straining.

Begin with a technique called the **Rising Breath** *(Uddhyana)*. It is very beneficial to health, strength, and brightness of mind, and it will help you master the movement needed for the Whirlwind.

Separate your feet and bend your knees slightly into a half-squat position, bracing yourself with your hands just above your knees. Tuck your chin into your throat. Begin by taking five deep and strong Belly Breaths (see page 101), to a count of three on both inhalation and exhalation, then breathe out forcefully and completely. Be sure all the air is expelled. Holding your breath out, suck in your abdominal muscles back toward your spine and up toward your diaphragm (21). Hold for just a moment, then release your stomach muscles, release your breath, breathe in, and relax. Stand up and rest until your breath returns to normal. Practice 3 repetitions.

When you feel relatively proficient in this movement, go on to the **Whirlwind** *(Nauli)*, which starts with a similar contraction that you then learn to move from side to side in your abdominal cavity. Begin in the same half-squat position (or seated), with chin tucked into your chest. Breathe in deeply, then breathe out forcefully and completely. Hold your breath out and suck in your abdominal muscles back toward your spine and up toward your diaphragm. Press down slightly on your left leg and you will feel the left side of your abdominal wall contract. Now press equally with both hands, and then with the right hand only. You will feel the abdominal contraction move across the front of your belly from left to right. Now equalize the pressure on your knees and slowly let your belly relax. Stand up straight and relax your breath and your entire body.

For daily practice, work up to 5 repetitions. Each repetition consists of left to center to right and back to center. Don't hold any of the positions for more than a few seconds. Always stand up and relax between repetitions. As you get stronger, you can do up to three cycles during each repetition. Be gentle with yourself. Rest immediately if you feel dizziness or discomfort.

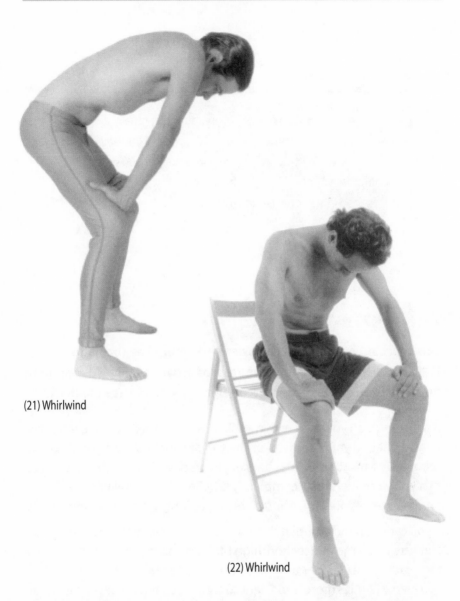

(21) Whirlwind

(22) Whirlwind

Note: If you have a lower back problem, or if you notice any discomfort in your mid-back or elsewhere in your back, begin this exercise seated in a chair instead (22). Sit on the edge of a sturdy chair with knees separated, and plant your feet firmly on the floor. Place hands on thighs with fingers pointed inward, as in the standing version. Proceed as instructed.

This exercise looks like a rest pose, but it is actually a very powerful technique for bringing all the parts of yourself into harmony. Gather yourself together internally as you strongly compress your body as much as you can without discomfort. Stop inner conversation. Try to stay silent in your mind.

BABY POSE (Virasan Var.)

Benefits: Limbers and relaxes lower back; improves circulation to the brain and pelvic region; improves reproductive and digestive systems functioning; improves respiration; helps to reduce a large stomach.

Kneel and sit on your feet with toes flat. Bend forward, keeping your hips on your feet, so your forehead or the top of your head rests on the floor. Bring your arms to your sides and let your elbows fall outward slightly so that your shoulders relax completely (23). Breathe naturally, through your nose, and relax your entire body. Hold for as long as you can comfortably.

If you cannot bend completely forward while keeping your hips on your feet due to a large midsection, high blood pressure, or extreme discomfort, just bend as far forward as you can or rest your head on folded arms or a pillow (24). It's more important to try to keep your hips on your heels than to rest your head on the floor. If your knees or hips are too stiff to do this exercise on the floor, you can sit in a straight chair with feet flat on floor and hips touching the back of the chair. Simply bend forward so that your head hangs over your knees and your arms hang loosely at your sides. Be sure to relax the back of your neck.

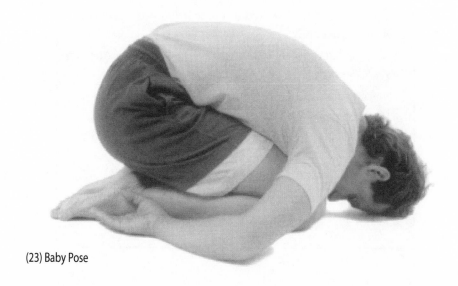

(23) Baby Pose

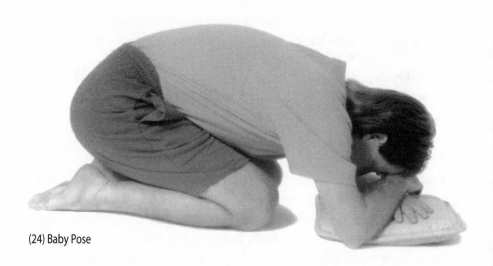

(24) Baby Pose

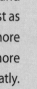

This sun pose is very effective in providing energy and health to the body. Practice it by visualizing the sun, just as you do with the standing sun pose. As you become more proficient in this exercise, you will become aware of more graceful movements, and your posture will improve greatly. When you are struggling with weight management, good posture can help you look and feel better instantly. This exercise has long-lasting effects on the straightness and lengthening of the spine. I practiced this exercise every day in the early years of my Yoga practice, and I grew three inches after the age of 35!

SEATED SUN POSE (Paschimottanasan)

Benefits: Stretches back of legs; limbers and strengthens lower back; massages internal organs.

Bring both legs straight out in front of you and flex your toes. Sit straight, breathe out with arms at your sides, then breathe in to a count of three as you raise your arms in a wide circle to the sides (25) and overhead. Press your palms together, look up, and stretch from the rib cage (26). Visualize the sun. Hold your breath in for a count of three.

Breathe out to a count of three as you bend forward, tucking your chin toward your chest. Grasp your ankles, bend your elbows, and pull your torso toward your legs (27). Remember to pull by bending your arms, not by pushing with your lower back. Hold your breath out for a count of three. If you are limber enough to reach your feet (and still bend your elbows), grasp your big toes as shown (28).

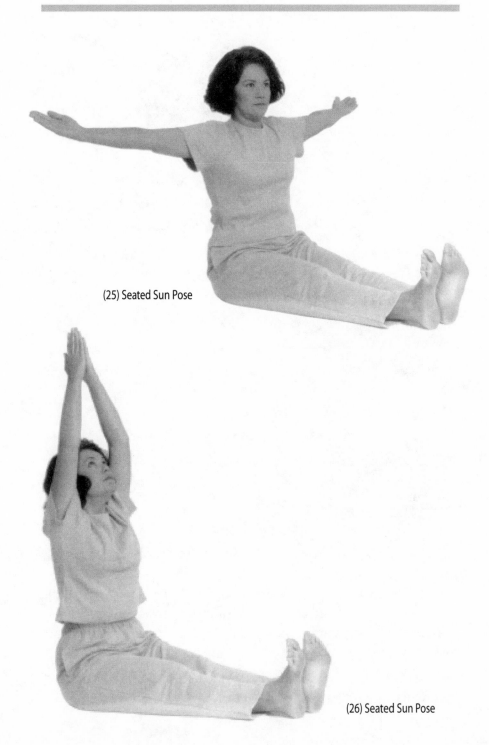

(25) Seated Sun Pose

(26) Seated Sun Pose

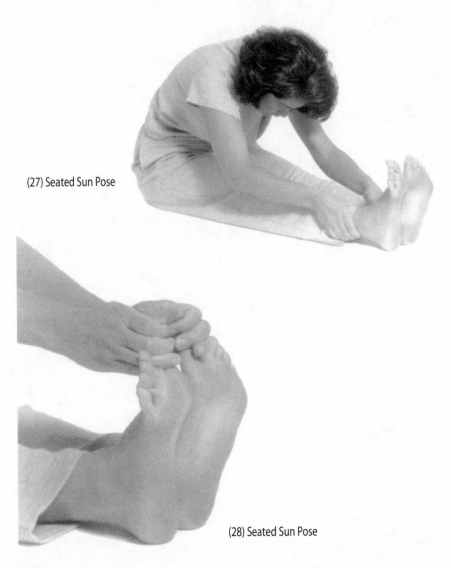

(27) Seated Sun Pose

(28) Seated Sun Pose

Release and breathe in to a count of three, bringing your arms to the sides and over your head again. Stretch and look up as before, and hold to a count of three. Breathe out, counting three, and bring your arms back down to your sides. Repeat 3 times.

This exercise may also be done sitting up in bed with legs outstretched, back supported by the headboard.

Along with good posture, a graceful carriage is another sign of a person who feels self-confident, healthy, and strong. This exercise promotes an easy, graceful walk and good balance. As you breathe and move according to the instructions, visualize your back straightening, your hips aligning, and the oxygen circulating throughout your body giving it renewed energy.

TORTOISE STRETCH (Kurmasan)

Benefits: Improves circulation to pelvic region through abdominal compression; stretches nerves and muscles in legs and ankles; limbers lower back; helps prevent prostate problems.

Separate your legs as far as possible and flex your toes. Straighten your back and breathe in to a count of three as you raise your arms in a wide circle to the sides and over your head (29). Hold for a count of three. Breathe out to a count of three as you bend forward and reach down over your right leg. Grasp your calf, ankle, or foot with both hands (30). If you can reach your toes easily, grasp the big toe with both hands as in the Seated Sun Pose (see p. 80). Hold your breath out for a count of three.

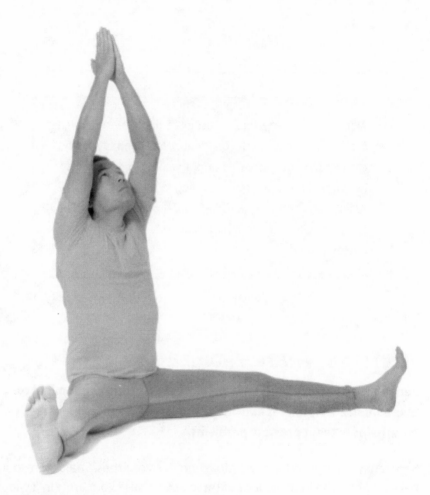

(29) Tortoise Stretch

Breathe in to a count of three as you raise your arms back over your head, then breathe out to a count of three as you lower your arms to your sides. Repeat 3 times to each side, then lean forward between your legs, grasp one leg or ankle with each hand and stretch forward as far as you can comfortably, relaxing your head and neck (31). Hold the position, breathing normally, for several seconds. Release and relax.

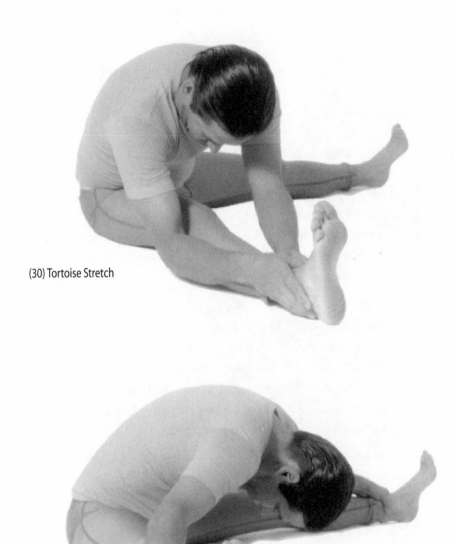

(30) Tortoise Stretch

(31) Tortoise Stretch

One of the ways you will know that you are making progress in your practice is when you stop thinking so much about the passing of time. Time loses its significance when you begin to live more in the present. My great teacher Lakshmanjoo said, "The past is dead, the future is not yet born." You will experience great strength and composure by practicing living in the moment. The Plank poses, which require some strength and balance, help you keep your mind on what you are doing. When you focus on your outstretched hand, keep your mind silent. Picture your body slim and supple as you breathe out.

The Plank pose provides vital weight-bearing exercise for increasing bone mass in the arms and shoulders. Regular weight-bearing exercise is especially important for women in order to prevent or slow the development of osteoporosis ("brittle bones"). Another important factor in the prevention of this disease is getting enough calcium. See Chapter 8 for more information about this vital nutrient.

PLANK POSE (Vasisthasan)

Benefits: Strengthens arms, shoulders, and neck; improves bone mass and circulation in upper body; strengthens back muscles.

From a hands-and-knees position, straighten your legs in back of you, supporting yourself on your toes and hands. Raise your hips and lower your shoulders until your body is in a straight line supported on your hands and feet. Shift your weight to your left arm and breathe in to a count of three as you lift your right arm straight in front of you (32).

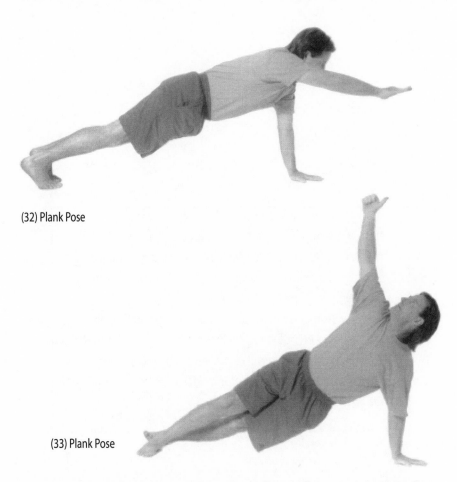

(32) Plank Pose

(33) Plank Pose

Focus your gaze on your outstretched hand. Hold your breath in for a count of three. Breathe out and release. Rest.

Still supporting yourself on your left arm, breathe in to a count of three as you bring your right arm to the side and up toward the ceiling (33), twisting your body to that side as well. Hold your breath in for a count of three, looking up at your right thumb. Breathe out to a count of three, bring the hand down to the floor, rest, and repeat the sequence on the opposite side. This exercise sequence is done only once on each side. Rest on your back for a minute or so before going on to the next exercise. Note: If you are not strong enough to do both positions on each side consecutively, do the first position (photo 32) on both sides, rest, then do the second position (photo 33) on both sides.

One of the places in our bodies that we tend to hold tension is the abdominal muscles, which affects breathing and digestion, among other processes. If you find yourself breathing very shallowly, clenching your teeth, or tightening your stomach muscles, you may find that this exercise will help you identify those common tension spots and relax them. This exercise will also strengthen your abdominal muscles so that you can better isolate them when you try the Whirlwind.

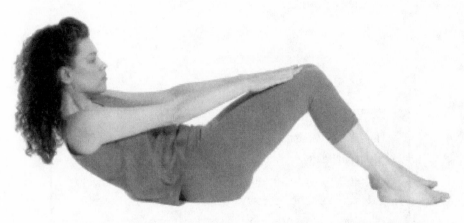

(34) Easy Sit-Up

EASY SIT-UP

Benefits: Strengthens abdominal muscles and upper back; relieves stomach and breath tension; massages internal organs.

This is an excellent exercise to use as a warmup to the Big Sit Up and other exercises that require abdominal strength. Lie on your back with your knees bent and your feet a comfortable distance apart. Straighten your arms and point your fingers toward your knees. Breathe in completely to a count of three as you raise your upper body using your abdominal muscles, sliding your hands up toward your knees (34). Hold for a count of three. Breathe out to a count of three as you return to your starting position. Repeat 3 times, working up to 15-20 repetitions.

Here is an exercise to try that allows you to attempt a position that may seem impossible at first. Most overweight people do not use the muscles needed for this exercise, and so it may seem hopelessly out of reach. Work into the exercise slowly. As a bonus, you will find that practicing this exercise every day works as a good appetite suppressant.

If your body shakes when you attempt this exercise, pay extra attention to your nutrition. Be sure you are eating foods rich in B vitamins for a healthy nervous system.

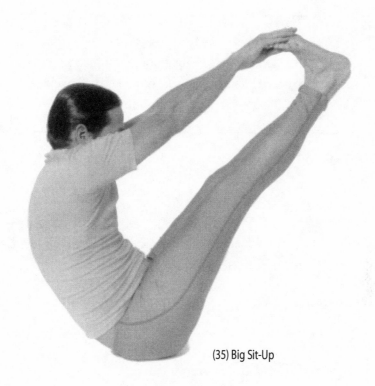

(35) Big Sit-Up

BIG SIT-UP (Supta Padangusthasan)

Benefits: Strengthens abdominal and leg muscles; improves balance and concentration; relieves constipation and urinary tract difficulties.

Lie on your back with arms over your head and legs together. Breathe in to a count of three as you lift your arms, legs, and upper body at the same time. Balancing on the end of your spine, reach to touch your toes, keeping your legs straight (35). Hold for a count of three or as long as you can, then relax and breathe out to a count of three as you lower yourself to the floor. Repeat twice more.

This exercise will make you feel like a dancer. Always move slowly, and use fantasy to imagine yourself supple, strong, slim, and graceful. Remember to fill your mind with silence as you hold the position. Do not talk to yourself.

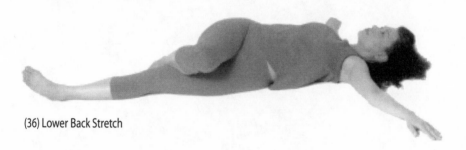

(36) Lower Back Stretch

LOWER BACK STRETCH

Benefits: Improves functioning of internal organs; improves circulation; strengthens and limbers the shoulders, back, and hip joints; helps to tone muscles in the midsection.

If you have spinal disk problems, check with your doctor before trying this exercise. Lie on your back with your legs together and arms stretched out to the sides, palms down. Breathe out, then breathe in to a count of three as you lift your right leg and hook the toe under your left leg. Breathe out to a count of three as you bend the lifted knee over your left leg as far as you can without straining (36), and hold the position and your breath for a count of three. Keep your shoulders and arms on the floor and keep your left leg very straight. Then breathe in to a count of three as you roll back, lifting your right leg straight to the ceiling and then slowly returning the leg to the floor. Repeat twice more on each side, alternating.

My teacher Rama told me that this is one of the best exercises for reducing body fat. It takes a bit of effort, but you will be proud of yourself for doing it. Be sure to rest completely at the end of the exercise. Each time you choose to try something that you are not sure you can do, you add to your self-confidence and strength. This is the Yogic ethic of Tolerance: choosing to do something that is a little difficult because you want to, not because someone else wants you to.

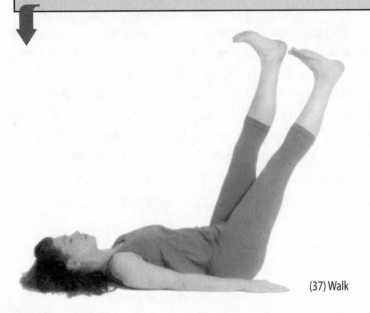

(37) Walk

WALK

Benefits: Reduces body fat; strengthens and tones legs, lower back, and abdomen.

Lie on your back with arms at your sides, palms down. Raise your legs straight up and flex your feet. "Walk" your legs back and forth (37), keeping your legs straight, for several seconds, breathing normally, then relax and lower your legs to the floor slowly.

Yoga exercises were designed to benefit the functioning of all the systems of the body: muscular, circulatory, respiratory, and glandular. The shoulder stand is one of the most efficient and powerful Yoga exercises, affecting all the body's systems. The inverted position stimulates circulation and respiration, and holding your legs erect strengthens the large muscle groups. The pressure of holding yourself upright on your shoulders improves bone mass in the shoulders and spine. The glandular system is particularly targeted due to the increased pressure on the thyroid gland, located in the neck. When you perform the exercise correctly, your chin presses into your neck, putting pressure on the thyroid. The shoulder stand is one of the best exercises for rapid weight loss because of this thyroid stimulation.

SHOULDER STAND (Sarvangasan)

Benefits: Stimulates thyroid and parathyroid glands; enhances function of all vital organs; relieves tension on heart and lungs; relaxes nervous system; removes fatigue; improves bone mass in upper spine.

If you have spinal disk problems in your neck or back, we suggest that you not do the full position; check with your doctor about trying a variation (photo 42) instead.

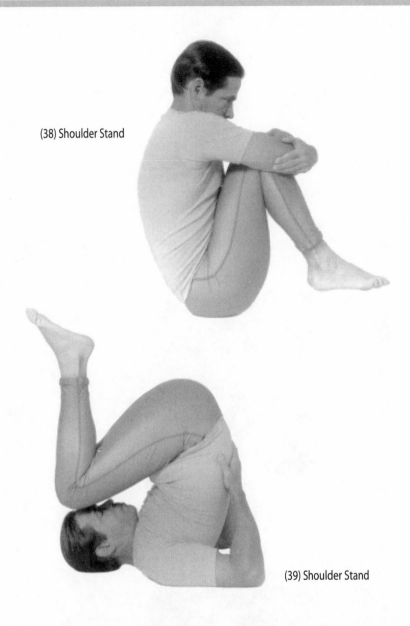

(38) Shoulder Stand

(39) Shoulder Stand

In a seated position with knees bent and arms around your knees (38), round your back and roll back and forth a few times, then roll back onto your shoulders, immediately supporting your back with your hands and keeping your knees bent and touching your forehead (39).

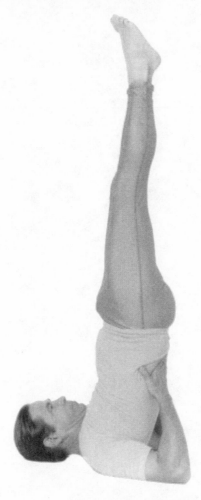

(40) Shoulder Stand

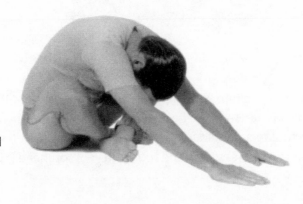

(41) Shoulder Stand

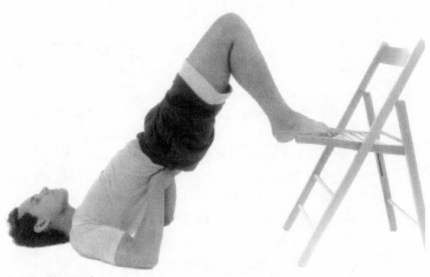

(42) Shoulder Stand

Slowly straighten your legs toward the ceiling and push your back straighter by using your hands (40). Stare at the spot between your big toes and breathe out. Hold your breath out for a count of three. Breathe in and relax your breath.

Bend your knees back to your forehead, supporting your back with your hands, then roll forward into a cross-legged position, reaching your head and arms forward (41). Breathe naturally as you rest for at least 10 seconds.

If you cannot do the full exercise, try this variation: Lie on your back with your hips pressed against a bed or chair and feet braced against the edge of the bed or chair. Breathe in completely. With arms at your sides, pressing down on the floor with your palms, breathe out to a count of three as you push against the bed or chair edge with your feet, lifting your hips and arching your back as much as possible without straining your neck. Bring your hands up to support your back (42). Hold for a count of three, then breathe in and relax back to your starting position. Repeat 3 times.

Yoga exercise places a great emphasis on strengthening the back muscles and spinal column, because your back is the support of your entire body. At least 20% of adults develop some kind of chronic back pain. Usually the cause can be traced to years of inactivity as well as unsafe lifting and carrying habits. The two exercises on these pages focus on strengthening the back muscles. The compression on the stomach acts as a stimulus to digestion. This exercise also helps to reduce appetite.

You are probably aware that eating a greater amount of fiber can help improve digestion. But did you also know that fiber also acts as an appetite suppressant? Because your body has to use more energy to break down the fiber, it takes a greater number of calories to process fiber-rich foods than foods that are low in fiber.

BOAT POSE (Poorva Navasan) & AIRPLANE POSE

Benefits: Strengthens spine; massages internal organs; improves breathing; strengthens shoulders, hips, and thighs.

Lying on your stomach, stretch your arms on the floor over your head and place your forehead on the floor. Breathe out. Breathe in to a count of three as you lift arms, legs, and head, looking up through your forehead (43). Hold for a count of three. Breathe out to a count of three as you return to your starting position. Repeat twice more.

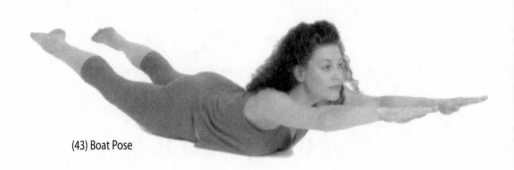

(43) Boat Pose

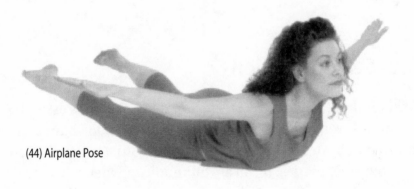

(44) Airplane Pose

Next, for the Airplane Pose, stretch your arms out to the sides, palms down. Breathe out. Breathe in to a count of three as you lift as before (44). Hold for a count of three. Breathe out to a count of three as you return to your starting position. Repeat twice more.

Chapter 4

Yoga Breathing Techniques for Weight Management

Your Seated Position

Establishing a comfortable, erect seated position is essential. You have several options; be assured that you don't have to get into a complicated cross-legged position in order to benefit from breathing techniques! If you are quite stiff, or when you are first learning the technique, just sit on the edge of a straight chair, with your feet flat on the floor or toes tucked under slightly. Do not lean against the back of the chair. Rest your hands on your knees. You may also do the exercises lying flat on the floor or on a bed until you get stronger.

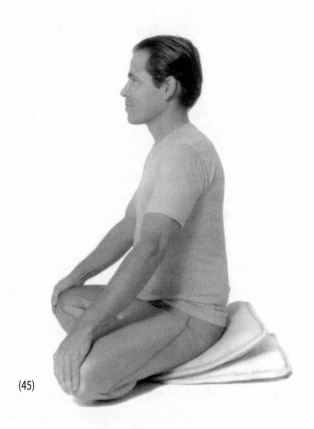

(45)

If your knees are fairly limber, you can try sitting on the floor, either kneeling or sitting cross-legged (45). If you sit cross-legged, be sure to use one or more firm cushions to raise your hips as shown in the photo. This will keep your lower back and stomach from becoming tense, which usually results in slouching. In order for the breathing techniques to work, your back must remain straight and relaxed.

Always Breathe Through Your Nose

Always inhale and exhale through your nose — never your mouth. My teacher Rama told me that breathing through the nose stimulates the glands in the head to supply a sweet nectar into the system. Breathing through your nose is important in regulating the speed of your breath and improving your concentration. It helps to focus on the sound of your breath. If you close your throat slightly, you will hear a steamlike sound as you breathe in and out. Concentrating on this sound will help you keep your attention on your breath.

If one side of your nose is blocked, try these techniques for opening it: If the right side is blocked, place your right fist in your left armpit and hold for a few minutes until the right side opens. Reverse the procedure to open the opposite side. Another method is to simply lie on your side for a few minutes: if the right nostril is blocked, lie on your left side, and vice versa. If neither of these techniques works, just do the best you can. Remember that although breathing through both nostrils equally is the ideal, you can still practice if your nose is partially blocked. The longer you practice Yoga, the more these passages will open.

When to Practice Breathing

When you are first starting to practice, do a few Complete Breath exercises at the beginning of your routine to help you get in the mood to practice and help you detach your mind from any cares or anxieties that you may be experiencing. Try to stop all inner conversation. Make the other breathing techniques in this section a part of your routine, preferably just before you lie down for meditation. You can also use breathing exercises — particularly the Complete Breath — any time of day to help calm stressful feelings you may be experiencing, to help fight cravings, or to change your thinking pattern. You can practice almost anywhere: lying in bed, in a waiting room at the bank or doctor's office, standing in line, or in the car while waiting for a light to change (please do not practice while actively driving).

Belly Breath

Place your hands loosely on your belly below your navel. Breath in through your nose and relax your belly as you imagine that you are filling your belly with air, expanding it and pushing your hands outward. This movement will relax all your internal organs and cause the diaphragm to drop to its fullest extent, allowing the air to reach the bottom section of your lungs. Breathe out now, through your nose, and slowly, consciously, contract your belly muscles, pushing in with your hands until all the air is out. Repeat several times. Do not hold your breath at any time. Remember: as you inhale the belly expands outward; as you exhale the belly contracts inward.

Complete Breath

In the Complete Breath, the movement of the Belly Breath is extended up into your ribs, where you expand the muscles between your ribs, and finally your chest, where you push air into the topmost sections of your lungs. Always breathe through your nose, and concentrate on the sound of the breath as described earlier.

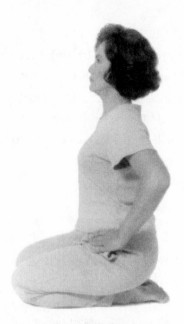
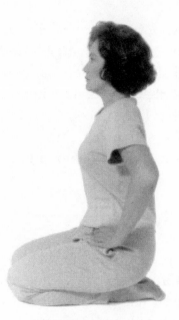

(46) Complete Breath   (47) Complete Breath

Place your hands on your belly and breathe out, trying not to slouch forward. Tighten your belly muscles to get as much air out as possible. Now begin to breathe in from the bottom up, letting your belly muscles relax so the air appears to fill your belly.

Continue to breathe in and feel the air filling the center part of your torso. Imagine the muscles between your ribs stretching so that your ribs expand in all directions, not just forward. Breathe in a little more and feel the air filling the very top sections of your lungs (46). Do not hold your breath, but gently start to breathe out, slowly, from the top down. First relax your chest, then let your ribs contract, and finally tighten your belly and push the last of the air out (47). Do not hold your breath at the bottom of the cycle either. Repeat the Complete Breath 3 to 10 times.

Depending on your current breath capacity, the complete cycle of the Complete Breath (one inhalation, one exhalation) may take 10 to 30 seconds. It is important to breathe in and out for approximately the same length of time. Most of us naturally breathe out longer than we breathe in. In the Complete Breath you are counteracting that tendency and learning to breathe more evenly.

Alternate Nostril Breath

The main purpose for this breathing technique is to balance the two halves of the body and the two bodies, the physical and emotional/spiritual, to give you full strength.

In a comfortable seated position or in a chair, curl the first and second fingers of your right hand inward, holding them down with the fleshy part of your thumb. The third and fourth fingers should remain extended. Close your right nostril with your thumb (48), and breathe in through the left nostril only. Hold for a count of three, then close the left nostril with your third and fourth fingers (49), open the right, and breathe out, hold for a count of three, then in again, through the right nostril. Continue alternating by breathing out, then in, through one side at a time. Repeat 5-10 times.

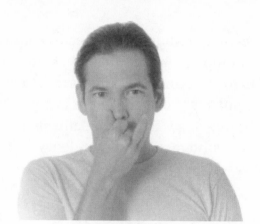

(48) Alternate Nostril Breath

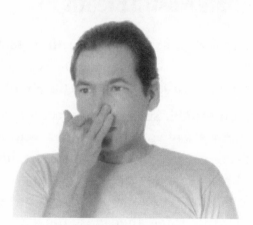

(49) Alternate Nostril Breath

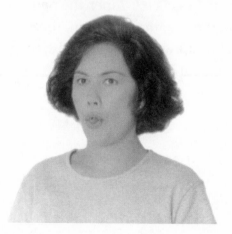

(50) Cooling Breath

The Cooling Breath *(Sitali)*

This technique has a cooling effect on the body; it also improves resistance to disease and enhances physical beauty.

In a comfortable seated position or in a chair, breathe out completely. Extend your tongue and curl the sides in (50). Breathe in slowly, then hold for a count of three. Exhale with mouth closed. Hold for a count of three. Make the inhalation and exhalation equal in length. Repeat 5-10 times.

Soft Bellows Breath *(Kapalabhati)*

This exercise tones and relaxes the muscles and nerves involved in respiration. It is an excellent preparatory technique for meditation because it focuses the mind very quickly. Its Sanskrit name literally means "shining skull," which refers to the power of this technique to stimulate the movement of energy through the body to the top of the head. In mythical language this implies that a lotus is opening at the top of the head as the physical and emotional bodies become charged with energy from respiration.

Sit comfortably in a cross-legged position with your hips raised on cushions, or sit on the edge of a chair with feet tucked under slightly. You may rest one hand on your belly to monitor the movement, or rest your hands on your knees or thighs. In this exercise, you breathe in the same way as the Belly Breath but slightly faster, so that you are moving the respiratory muscles a little more strongly. Breathe in for a count of three, then out for a count of three, without holding your breath either at the top or the bottom. The inhalation and exhalation should be equal in length. One cycle equals three inhalations and exhalations. Start with three cycles (nine breaths), and work up to eleven cycles (thirty-three breaths). At the end of each cycle, relax your breath and rest for at least a count of three. You will find that when you are able to do this exercise correctly, it is impossible to carry on inner conversation while you are practicing.

Chapter 5

Yoga Meditation for Weight Management

Your Meditation Position

In meditation you will be practicing "thinking nothing," which will lead you to silence. To quiet your mind successfully, your physical body must be completely relaxed, and you cannot relax if you are straining to maintain an uncomfortable seated position. For this reason, we strongly suggest that you begin to learn meditation lying flat (51). That way, you can forget about your body while you focus on quieting your thoughts and feelings.

If you are unable to lie on your back, you may sit in a chair as long as your back is straight — this is very important for meditation practice. Eventually, as you proceed in practice, you can try a comfortable seated position such as one of those described for the breathing exercises in Chapter 4 (see pages 98-99).

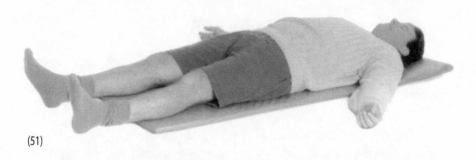

(51)

Clothing and Equipment

Lie on the blanket or mat that you use for Yoga practice; if it is too short for your entire body, rest your head on it. Do not use a pillow under your head unless you have to. It is important not to put pressure on the back of your neck. If your lower back feels tense, you can place a few pillows under your knees. Wear your exercise clothes, and put on socks to keep your feet warm. Wrap your upper body with a shawl or blanket; your body temperature will drop as your body relaxes and your mind fills with silence, and you don't want to become chilled.

Protect Yourself from Disturbance

Ask family members not to interrupt you during your meditation time, and make sure pets are in another area. Turn off your telephone. Keep your practice space quiet and secure; sudden noises or intrusions can be quite shocking when you are completely relaxed and intensely quiet. Do not play music during any part of Yoga practice, because you want to experience your own thoughts and feelings free of outside influences. Silence is important.

Your Meditation Experience

Meditation is the key to bringing your two bodies, the physical and the emotional, together in harmony. If you practice a few minutes of meditation every day, along with a few exercises, it won't be long before you start to experience the satisfying power of operating as a whole person. You will quickly notice, with practice, that you become extremely intuitive.

Meditation is not concentrating on your breath, or a sound, or anything else; it is simply no thought. One of the best ways to explain the meditation experience is that you simply try to stop talking to yourself. In the beginning, you may notice just a few seconds of quietness after you stop thinking one thought before another thought slips in. Meditation is a continuous process of increasing awareness. You start out in quietness, then before you know it your mind is full of plans, memories, anxieties, and other thoughts. Then you remember to stop talking to yourself, you are quiet for a while, and then the whole process begins again. Try to remember what it feels like when you are not thinking. Eventually you will be able to recreate that feeling at will, and that will help you maintain the quiet feeling for longer periods of time.

Some people fall asleep when they first begin learning how to meditate. This is perfectly natural, and you will experience a very restful type of sleep. If you are practicing in the morning and are afraid that you will sleep too long, try not to use an alarm clock, because the loud noise will startle you and upset your system. Simply tell yourself mentally, before you begin your meditation, that you wish to meditate for a certain length of time — say, 10 minutes — and you will find that you naturally "wake up" after that time has passed. I suggest that you begin by meditating for 10 minutes daily, and work up to 20 or 30 minutes if you wish.

Complete Relaxation Procedure

Lie on your back with your arms at your sides, palms up. Let your fingers curl naturally, and let your feet fall slightly outward. This is called the Corpse Pose. This complete relaxation procedure will take 5 to 10 minutes. The idea is to completely relax every bone, muscle, and nerve in your body so that you can forget about your body while you meditate. A cassette tape on which I lead you through the entire relaxation/meditation procedure is available from the American Yoga Association; see Resources.

Read over the following directions and then close your eyes and begin relaxing. You will be focusing your attention quietly on each part of your body, visualizing each part in turn without moving any part of your body except your breath. Simply tell yourself to relax each body part in your mind.

Start with your face. Gently and calmly bring all of your attention to your forehead. Feel all of the muscles in your forehead. Let them relax so they feel loose.

Become aware of your eyes. Are they tense and jumpy? The eyes are usually the most difficult body part to relax, so just let them loosen and float in the sockets. Let all tension and movement in the eyes stop. Move on to your lips, teeth, and all the muscles of the jaw, mouth, and throat. Let your tongue relax in your mouth, and say to yourself, "I don't have to speak for a few minutes." Feel all the skin on your face become loose. Let your scalp relax and imagine your ears drooping toward the floor. Your eyes may continue to jump around a little, but after regular practice you will be able to relax them more and more.

Now relax your shoulders, arms, and hands. Feel as if your arms were hollow. Let all the muscles of the shoulders settle loosely on the floor. Move down into your elbow joints and imagine you can see and feel the bones. Relax and loosen them. Do the same with your forearms, wrists, and right into your hands and fingers, making them hollow and loose. Relax your fingers completely as though they were empty gloves lying on the floor.

Silently move your attention, like a tiny, warm relaxing beam of light, into your chest and, for a few moments, just observe the air moving in and out of your lungs. Feel your heart beating softly and rhythmically. Notice your belly rising and falling as you breathe. Do not try to speed up or slow down your breathing. Instead, just picture your lungs. Then take in a gentle breath of air, and, just as though you are sighing, let the breath out and relax your lungs. Take in another deep, gentle breath, sigh it out, and feel your heart relaxing also. Then let go of your breathing altogether and relax all tension or effort in your breathing. Observe your belly and try to relax the squeezing effort as you breathe out. Each time you exhale, make your breath as relaxed as possible so that you are exerting almost no effort to breathe.

Now move your attention down into your legs, picturing them hollow, just as you did with your arms. Loosen and relax your thighs, hip sockets, and groin. Relax your knee joints and feel as though your lower legs are also hollow and empty, all the way into your toes. Imagine that your feet are empty — nothing inside, not even any bones. Feel your toenails relax and loosen.

Move up inside your empty feet, legs, and thighs, and bring your attention to the base of your spine. As you move upward through your waist area, relax any sign of tension so that your entire spine feels rubbery and loose. Feel your spine and all of its joints all the way up to the base of your skull. Spend a little extra time at the back of your neck. This common tension site needs extra attention. Imagine you can look right down inside your spinal column as though your spine were a rope dangling down into a dark well. Relax your spine so much that it feels as loose as that rope.

Next, concentrate on moving inside your head. Bring your attention back to your face to check whether or not your face is tense. Relax your eyes even more now, and let them float almost as though you can't feel them move at all.

Recheck the three main tension areas. 1) Is your breathing relaxed? 2) Are your eyes and facial muscles relaxed? 3) Is the back of your neck relaxed? Your body will eventually feel as if it were just an empty shell with no tension anywhere. The only movement will be your heart and your breathing, but they also will be very relaxed. Now relax the entire inside of your head. Feel your brain quietly settling inside your head with no effort or strain — just quiet and still.

Here is a summary of the relaxation steps:

1. *Relax your face and eyes.*

2. *Relax and empty your arms and hands.*

3. *Relax your lungs and heart.*

4. *Relax your belly and breathing.*

5. *Relax and empty your legs and feet, especially your thighs and knees.*

6. *Relax and loosen your back, shoulders, and neck.*

7. *Relax the inside of your head.*

8. *Recheck the three major tension areas: 1) your face and eyes; 2) your breathing; 3) the back of your neck.*

Meditation

Now you are ready to meditate. Start your meditation period by thinking of the sound "Om" (pronounced "ohm"). This word is a sound formula that has a specific effect on the mind when it is repeated or heard. "Om" is the oldest and most basic sound in classical Yoga. It has been said that if you could hear the subtle humming sound of the collective atomic structure of your own body and mind, that sound would most resemble the sound Om.

The Om sound of classical Yoga has been adopted and used in a religious way by nearly every religion of the Eastern world. However, in classical Yoga, the sound Om is used to center and focus the mind, and is not meant to indicate any particular religious concept or deity. Its purpose is to empty the mind except for the sound itself, leading finally to complete silence.

When you practice meditation, you will probably find that your experience of silence will be deeper and more refreshing if you repeat the sound "Om" to yourself several times at the beginning of your meditation session. Then simply stop talking to yourself in your mind. Try to stop all inner conversation. Don't force it; meditation is a process, not something that can be mastered overnight. Treat your daily meditation session like a game; see how long you can be still before a thought interrupts you. Some days you will be able to be still for a long time; other days it will be difficult to stop talking to yourself or even stop thinking even for a second. Just keep trying every day and focus on the refreshing, quiet feeling that stays with you after your meditation session.

Eventually you will notice that this feeling will accompany you throughout your day. All you have to do is remember the feeling and it will be there. Many students tell me that their daily meditation period is as refreshing as taking a short nap. It is a tremendous help to concentration.

After Meditation

How you come out of meditation is as important as how you relax into it. If you get up too quickly, you may feel irritable or upset. When you open your eyes, before you start to move around, lie still for a few minutes longer thinking about the sensations, feelings, and thoughts that you experienced during your meditation period. Then increase your breathing a little to start reactivating your body and consciousness. At first, when you start to move your hands and arms, they may feel a little like wood since they've become so utterly relaxed. Make fists of your hands; then release them. Keeping your legs straight on the floor, flex your feet back toward your chin and then point them away. Do this a few times. Stretch your arms and legs like a cat does when it awakens from a nap. As you move toward your normal activities, you will feel refreshed, alert, and recharged with new energy and a clear mind.

Chapter 6

Yoga Fantasy Techniques for Weight Management

If you have a weight imbalance, you find yourself spending a lot of energy on the problem. It is always on your mind, and it affects all the decisions and relationships in your life. Those lucky few who never worry about their weight seldom understand the continual drain of personal power that weight imbalance demands. A loss of confidence accompanies all your activities, as well as loss of a pleasing self-image. If you don't believe that you look your best, you seldom find the courage to compete in daily life activity. It takes a brave person to live a full life in spite of an appearance that deviates from the norm. Yet a pleasing appearance depends not so much on the external form as on the support from the inner body. The self-confidence that brings this about can come from the practice of Yoga, particularly through the use of Fantasy.

Fantasy will help you adjust to your new shape and size as you progress with our program. The choice of what clothing to buy or wear, for example, is sometimes a shock because what worked for you before is now passé. The physical body invents clever ways to keep its appearance from changing; you can counteract that tendency by trying to see yourself in your new body look each day in Fantasy. Once I had a student who lost a great deal of weight successfully. The classroom where we met for our Yoga classes had a passageway between two pillars that my student had always avoided when he was heavy because it was uncomfortable to squeeze through. After he had lost the weight and clearly could fit through the space with ease, he still avoided it. When I asked him why, he said, "Oh, I'm much too big to fit through there!" Obviously he had not yet formed a new image of himself to match his new size.

Many times, self-destructive behavior is hidden in our vision of ourselves. Constant effort must be made to change your vision of yourself to what you want it to be, not a vision that portrays you as a victim. Often, in their zeal to begin getting results, people rush into a harsh discipline, which upsets both bodies, setting the stage for the kind of vengeful reactions described previously. I suggest that you do not force a quick and ruthless change of eating habits upon yourself. Start slowly, and create a gradual change of lifestyle that allows your physical and emotional bodies to get used to the new routine, making it much more likely that you will continue. Most importantly, every day practice a Fantasy vision of yourself as you wish to be. This is the key to establishing that new vision as you continue to change your behavior.

How to Practice Fantasy Exercises

In the following pages I will teach you some easy Fantasy techniques to practice as part of your daily Yoga routine. The first
time you practice a Fantasy exercise, set aside 10 to 15 minutes
in a private place where you won't be disturbed. After you are
familiar with the techniques, you can try practicing them while
walking (see Chapter 7), or you can incorporate them into many
other activities of daily life. An excellent time to practice Fantasy is just before you go to sleep at night. Note: Please do not
practice Fantasy exercises while driving, operating dangerous
machinery, or any other activity that requires your full attention
for safety reasons. Consider your focus on safety at those times
to be a practice of the Yogic ethic of Nonviolence toward yourself, and remember to practice your Fantasy exercises at another
time.

Creating a Vision of Yourself

Start by looking at yourself in a mirror, preferably full-length.
Look at yourself for a minute or two, reminding yourself of all
the things that you have said to yourself before about what you
like or do not like about yourself. Now sit or lie down in a comfortable position and close your eyes. Take a few deep complete
breaths and then let your breath return to normal. Let your entire body go limp and relaxed. Now, in your mind, imagine yourself standing in front of the mirror again, but this time, visualize
yourself the way you would like to be. If your goal is to lose
weight, picture yourself thinner. If you are also working on posture and muscle tone, picture yourself standing straight and

proud. Don't limit yourself to physical attributes; picture yourself confident, poised, radiant with good health and strength — every desirable quality that you can think of. Hold that vision in your mind for as long as you can in silence. Then take another deep breath, let it out, and notice how you feel. Tell yourself how you feel, and remind yourself that you can recall that feeling whenever you need it or want it. Open your eyes and go about your day with new energy.

The "I Love You" Meditation Technique

Throughout this book, I talk about the importance of self-confidence in your weight management program. This technique is one of the best ways I know to give yourself the confidence you need and want. It is easy to do, and once you learn the technique, I urge you to use it throughout the day in different ways. For example, one of my students stands in front of the mirror every morning drying his hair. All the time his blow-dryer is on, he repeats "I love you" to his reflection in the mirror, with no other thought in his mind, until his hair is dry. He says that this simple practice has changed his life.

This technique is a complement to, not a substitute for, daily meditation practice. You will need to set aside about 15-20 minutes for this technique. Try it just before bed for a restful, refreshing sleep. Prepare yourself just as if you were going into meditation: lie on your back on your blanket, keep warm, and protect yourself from disturbances.

Start with what may seem a strange technique: Pump your arms and legs vigorously as if you were riding a bicycle, so that your whole body is moving. Laugh out loud and be as silly as you can imagine for about 30 seconds! This exercise will stimulate the brain chemicals that contribute to feelings of well-being. Then relax your body, settle in to your meditation position, and let your breath relax.

Bring your attention to your forehead. Breathe in, saying "I love you" to yourself. Do the same as you breathe out. Repeat several times: breathe in "I love you" and breathe out "I love you." Breathe in and hold for a moment. Imagine the feeling "I love you" spreading throughout your brain in a beautiful, warm, wet, perfumed essence. Breathe out "I love you."

Relax completely. Let your breath relax. Hold that feeling. Then, for a few more minutes, continue saying "I love you" each time you breathe in and out. As you breathe in and hold your breath for a moment, think to yourself, "Whom do I love?" Breathe out and say "I love you." Breathe in and hold again; think: "Who loves me?" Now think to yourself: "My breath loves me." Breathe out. "My breath loves me." The breath is inside you. It loves you. Breathe in and think "I'm holding my breath — it loves me." Breathe out and think "I have released my breath — it still loves me." Take a deep breath, always through your nose. Breathe in: "My breath loves me." Breathe out: "My breath is gone now but it still loves me."

Relax completely. Visualize the inside of your head and your body. Think of the breath commingled with love. Oxygen is flowing through your arteries and heart and every part of you because you can't live without your breath. Visualize this loving breath inside your body. Are there any blocks keeping it from moving where it wants to go? Visualize this feeling of love and breath removing any kind of constriction, moving easily and sweetly throughout your body.

Bring the feeling to your forehead. Think "I love you — my breath is in my forehead." Relax your forehead. Now think of this feeling of love spreading to your eyes — you can almost see it! Relax your eyes and let the breath of love simply swim out into the rest of your face. Feel this breath of love in your nose, because it breathes for you. Every time you breathe in, breathe "I love you." Every time you breathe out, breathe "I love you." Let the breath of love flow freely so that your face melts with love. Let your mouth and throat relax, thinking "I love you" as you breathe.

Let your neck relax now so you have no constriction that will stop the breath from moving. Love comes in with your breath — relax. Love goes out with your breath — relax. Drop your collarbone toward the floor and say "I love you." Let the ends of your shoulders drop. Do the same with your arms; let them relax; feel that they are fully supported by this breath of love. Rest your arms in love. Relax your wrists. Let your hands be totally relaxed in love. You're vulnerable. You don't care. You can't lose love. Breath comes in and it goes out, and love is still there. Relax your fingers, letting them curl slightly, like a baby's hand when it is asleep.

Move your attention to your chest. Be aware that you are taking a breath into your heart: "I love you." Breathe it out with love. Breathe into your lungs: "I love you." Breathe out "I love you." Now relax your entire chest. Let your breath relax in love. Become aware that this breath is love. You're not making it happen; it's happening because it loves you.

Breathe in and think of your stomach. Breathe out and say "I love you" as you relax your stomach. Relax your abdomen, thinking: "I love you. I love you the way you are." Feel the breath of love move through your hip joint. Warm, liquid, lubricating, beautiful — perfectly balanced and poised. Say "I love you" to your hips and relax them. Let the large bones in the top of your legs sink toward the floor; you don't have to hold them up. You love them. They love you. You can't lose love. Relax your legs in love. Relax your knees and ankles and think "I love you." Think to your feet "I love you." Relax your feet.

Picture yourself just simply floating; completely supported on this breath, this love. Bring your attention up to the back of your hips and the base of your spine. Open it up like a flower. Say "I love you." Don't fight it. Let it flow easily, smooth and quiet. Relax the back of your shoulder blades. Let your back get soft. Love is supporting you. "I love you, back." The back of your neck relaxes. Think to yourself, "I love you. I love you." Then you reach your brain, your hair, all soft and supported, resting in love, in breath.

Breathe in and think love. Breathe out — love is still there. Think of your brain floating in a pool of this love. Now make it totally quiet. Then simply say to yourself, "I love you." Bring your mind to your forehead and think nothing. Hold this feeling of quietness. If you feel any other thought coming in, make sure that it says "I love you." Transpose any thought to "I love you" and go back to thinking nothing. Think nothing as long as you can. Stop talking to yourself. Become silent internally.

Rest quietly like this for about 10 minutes, then slowly stretch, take a deep breath and let it out, and think about how you feel. Rest on your side or stomach for a few minutes enjoying the feeling before you get up. Move slowly back into your normal attitudes and lifestyle with a new vision of yourself.

During this exercise, it is important to note who is loving you. Regular practice of the "I love you" technique will open expression channels for love from your inner emotional body. It gives attention to the body that will replace the loss of extra food. Every time you take something away from the physical body it must be offered a replacement for what it has lost or it will take vengeance on the emotional body. Similarly, if you deny expression to the emotional body, it will take vengeance on the physical. The goal is to find a happy balance where neither body fears the other. Fantasy is the best way to achieve this balance, and the "I love you" technique is the basis for this practice of providing daily attention to the body in ways other than the intake of food. A cassette tape of this technique is available from the American Yoga Association; see Resources.

The Hall of Doors

This technique is very helpful for concentrating on a particular problem or concern. For example, suppose interaction with a particular person is so stressful that you always overeat after you see this person. Using this technique, you can practice those stressful interactions and perhaps change the way you respond. Another example is fear of failure, something that nearly everyone who begins a new weight-loss program faces in some measure. This technique will help you face your fear and build the strength to overcome it.

This Fantasy exercise requires a concentrated period of about 5-10 minutes. Lie down on your back on your mat with your arms at your sides, legs together, and eyes closed. This is called the Corpse Pose. Do not use a pillow behind your head in order to avoid pressure on the back of your neck. You can also do this exercise sitting in a chair as long as your back is straight. Stay warm. Completely relax your body as if you were about to meditate (see page 110).

Begin your Fantasy exercise by bringing your inner attention to your forehead. Imagine that you are looking down a long hallway. There are several doors leading off this central hallway: some to the left, some to the right. Picture the hallway in every detail: the color of the walls, whether the floor is carpet, tile, or wood; the color of and type of hardware on the doors; the lighting in the hallway — invent all these small details in your Fantasy. Make it complete in your mind before you enter it.

Now before you walk down the hall, protect yourself by covering your entire body with armor. Imagine the most beautiful, heroic suit that you can, with all of the details, such as the color and weight of the armor, the type of helmet and gloves, the boots, and the fastenings. When your body is completely protected with armor, then create a beautiful sword of your own design and take it in your hand.

The reason for all this protection is that, in Fantasy, you are exploring the unknown realm of your unconscious. Although everything in your mind is part of you, much of it will seem unfamiliar, and it might even feel a bit frightening at first. Our conscious mind often feels anxiety about anything that is unknown; the symbolic protection of the armor and sword that you create in your mind lets you enter and observe your Fantasy world protected and without fear.

When you have a clear picture of your armor and sword, imagine yourself entering the hallway. Each door has the name of some problem or concern written on it. Choose one of the doors, put your hand on the knob, and open it. Stand protected by your armor and sword, and simply observe what is in that room. Realize that you can step back and shut the door anytime you wish. I suggest that at first you try to observe for about a minute before leaving the room. When you decide to leave, shut the door, walk back down the hall, remove your armor, and observe yourself resting in the Corpse Pose. Give yourself plenty of time to change your orientation from the Fantasy experience back to resting. Then, for a few minutes, think about what you have discovered.

The names on the various doors in your hallway can correspond to the concerns that are uppermost in your mind as you work with your weight management program. Some examples are fear of attack, self-hate, anxiety about your chances of success, difficulty in a relationship, pressure at work, and so on. Do not try to open all the doorways in one session; one at a time is enough! Try a new one each week.

Sometimes students tell me that they feel like quitting in frustration, saying that they never see anything when they open the doors in their Fantasy. Usually I find that these people are afraid to try, which tells me that the obstacle confronting them is unusually difficult. If you find yourself in this position, simply continue with the Fantasy exercise until you begin to enjoy some success. Probably you have never attempted to communicate with your unconscious mind before. If you continue to do the technique, eventually something will appear. I have never known a student who didn't eventually find something behind the door.

This technique will work best if you can practice it daily for at least a week. You will quickly experience great improvement in your concentration and your ability to deal with daily problems.

Most of all, however, regular practice of this exercise allows the hidden, unseen experience of your inner body to show itself to you. It is no longer something that you just feel; it takes shape, and you are fully protected to face it and respond to it. When you have mastered the technique, you will find that you can use it as an immediate solution to whatever problems are hindering your progress in your weight management program.

Chapter 7

Walking Contemplation for Weight Management

Whether you are trying to lose weight or simply avoid gaining weight, a regular exercise program is a must. Exercise not only burns calories, but also helps your body maintain general health. Regular exercise feels good, too. When you are active, your body circulates more blood to your brain, bringing it more oxygen and releasing the chemicals called endorphins that contribute to feelings of well-being.

In this chapter, I am going to teach you how to incorporate regular exercise into your daily life as part of your Yoga routine for Weight Management. If you can get into the habit of doing your Yoga routine every day, you will improve your concentration and your health, and you will enjoy exercise more. It won't become boring. Most importantly, you will lose weight faster and tend to keep it off.

You can practice this technique while walking, swimming, or riding a stationary bicycle. I have chosen to focus on these three forms of exercise because they are easy to do and, more importantly, they are not dangerous to do while your attention is elsewhere. Walking and cycling also are quite effective at changing your metabolic rate. They are low-impact — much easier on your joints than running or other high-impact sports. I do not recommend cycling on the street, simply because you will have to pay too much attention to traffic and other hazards to be able to concentrate fully on the technique. If you are an experienced exerciser used to running or jogging, you can try adapting this technique for use on a treadmill.

Who Exercises?

If you are overweight and live in the Midwest, you are more likely to exercise than if you live in a Southern state, according to a 1998 survey. The survey also found that more education means more exercise as well: college-educated overweight people are more likely to exercise than those without a high school diploma. Slightly more men than women in the survey said that they exercise regularly.

Bhairavi Mudra

This technique, which I am calling "walking contemplation," is based on an ancient Yogic technique called Bhairavi Mudra (bye-RAH-vee MOO-dra). Both of my great teachers used to use this technique while walking in the mountains of Kashmir. Here is a rough translation of the verse that describes the technique:

> *Bhairavi mudra is a pose in which the eyes are open externally without blinking, but the attention is turned to the inner essential Self. Though the eyes are open, the aspirant sees nothing of the external world.*

This is a bit like meditating with your eyes open. Think of the "inner essential Self" as the feeling of stillness that you experience while meditating (see Chapter 5). While you are walking (or swimming or cycling), simply turn your mind inward and try to reexperience the feeling of stillness. Stop talking to yourself internally.

Try to turn all your senses inward as well. For instance, you see the roses in your neighbor's garden as you pass by. While practicing Walking Contemplation, you try not to name the flowers or let your thoughts turn to your own garden; you just experience the sensation of seeing the colors and shapes and move on as you feel stillness inside. You may hear birds singing, or other noises; try not to name the noise or look for it, but simply walk on with your attention turned to inner silence. In other words, try not to use language in the experience.

You will find this to be a continual process. Just as in the concentrated meditation period that you do as part of your daily Yoga routine (see Chapter 5), you will find that sometimes it is easier to feel stillness than at other times. In the beginning you may be able to focus on stillness only for a few seconds at a time.

The Ethic of Nonhoarding

The practice of Bhairavi Mudra will sharpen your awareness of the subtle aspects of hoarding. Whenever you name an object that you see — flowers, fence, etc. — you are in a sense owning that object. In Walking Contemplation, you are trying to reduce that outward reach of your mind in order to focus on the feeling of stillness. The experience of that stillness, where "names and forms" (*namarupa*, in Sanskrit) leave the mind, is one aspect of the ethical practice of Nonhoarding.

Eventually, something that you see or hear or remember starts the thinking process — and inner talking — again. Whenever you notice yourself thinking about something else, gently bring your attention back to stillness. Don't force it, and try not to judge yourself. Look at it like a game that you are playing with yourself. See how long you can do it.

When I first began this practice, I tried it while walking through a department store and was overwhelmed by the seemingly infinite number of recognitions, categorizations, and even judgments that my brain was capable of producing. It was as if the huge number of objects surrounding me were all demanding a response from me, which was distracting and upsetting, even to the point of often becoming sick to my stomach. If you find that you are always tired after a shopping trip, perhaps you are experiencing this also, and you might find the technique of Bhairavi Mudra helpful. After long practice of this technique myself, I have found that the chaos of these earlier adventures is much reduced, and trips to the mall are a lot more peaceful.

If you find that it is too hard to focus on stillness at first, or if you just want a change of pace, you can substitute other subjects for contemplation. Here are a few suggestions:

• **Focus on Nonviolence, or some other ethic:** Use your exercise time to focus on how you can practice Nonviolence in yourself, such as stopping self-critical thoughts, counteracting "ugly fits" when you look in the mirror, eating sensibly, and so on. (If you are interested in finding out more about this and other ethics of Yoga, they are discussed at length in my book *Yoga of the Heart*; see Resources.)

In other sessions, focus on practicing Nonviolence toward others, such as a spouse, child, or co-worker; think about some ways in which you may have acted in a hurtful way toward the person, and mentally rehearse future interactions in which you respond nonviolently.

• **Practice the "I Love You" technique:** While you are exercising, practice the "I Love You" technique in your mind (see page 118), repeating the phrase on your breath and carrying it throughout your body just as if you were lying down.

• **Watch your breath:** In the same way that you concentrate on stillness, concentrate on your breath. Do not change your breath; simply watch it. Listen to the sound of your breath as you walk. (See page 100 for more on the sound of your breath.) It helps to talk to your breath: Encourage it and praise it.

Beginning Your Exercise Program

Following are some tips to make the exercise portion of this technique more effective. Although these instructions focus primarily on walking, you can easily adapt them for swimming and cycling. I've added some particular recommendations for swimming and cycling where appropriate.

Start Gradually

The most common mistake people make in beginning a new exercise program is overdoing it, demanding too much of muscles that are not accustomed to being worked and creating stress by making too drastic a lifestyle change all at once. By gradually incorporating small increments of exercise time into your daily schedule, you will start looking forward to the feelings of relaxation and stress relief that exercise brings rather than seeing it as "one more thing I have to do today." If you start slowly, and gradually build up your exercise time, you will be more likely to enjoy it and keep it up as part of your new healthy lifestyle.

I find that people often overdo in the beginning, not out of naïve overenthusiasm but actually in order to defeat the effort. As I discussed in previous chapters, if the inner emotional body is not acknowledged and nourished, it will do everything it can to return the body to its previous state. The inner emotional body sabotages our plans with an initial euphoria that urges us to do more than we can sustain, making it more likely that we will overdo and eventually quit altogether. If you notice this tendency in yourself, try to restrain the impulse to do too much, and reassure your inner body with statements such as, "Little by little, I am changing my vision of myself. I will love the way I look and feel as I gradually create new enjoyable habits of diet and exercise." Another way to acknowledge your inner body is through fantasy: Try the Fantasy exercise of the Hall of Doors, picture your frightened inner body in one of the rooms, and then console it, "sweet-talk" it, in fantasy, and develop a closer communication with it.

Whether you are very sedentary and unaccustomed to any exercise, or someone who is more active but wanting to adopt a more regular fitness program, I recommend this single goal for the first two weeks: Get out the door and walk (or swim, or cycle) for a comfortable period of time four times each week. Don't worry about time, mileage, or pacing; simply get used to practicing the contemplation exercise while you are exercising. It may be 5 minutes, it may be 20 minutes; just enjoy the benefits of taking care of yourself. Give your body a chance to enjoy a little exercise without taking the approach of a stern taskmaster.

Keep in mind that the goal is to develop a new lifestyle; a new way of looking at what is important to health and well-being each day. Although I recommend exercising four days per week in the beginning, set your goal on attaining at least five days of exercise per week eventually, and preferably seven days. If you start slowly and progress gradually, you will enjoy exercising so much that you won't want to miss a day!

Beginning in week three, add 5 minutes to your exercise time each week (never add more than 5 minutes per week). In week four, take 5 minutes to warm up as part of your allotted time, pick up the pace a little during your main exercise period, then add 5 minutes for cool down (see below). Continue adding 5 minutes per week until you reach a total of 40 minutes (5 minutes warmup, 30 minutes brisk activity, 5 minutes cool down) four or more days per week. See Resources for some excellent books on walking, cycling, and swimming if you'd like to refine your technique or add to your program.

Note: You don't have to exercise all at once to reap the benefits of exercise. As long as the exercise is vigorous, you can achieve the same results in three 10-minute segments throughout the day as in 30 minutes of sustained exercise. You can also add even more exercise time to your day by doing such things as:

- parking at the far end of the lot and walking briskly into the store or work.

- taking the stairs instead of the elevator.

- walking the dog at a good pace.

Just remember that your total time spent in briskly paced activities each day should add up to at least 30 minutes (not counting warm-up and cool down time).

Warm Up

Always begin your exercise session by walking slowly for 5-10 minutes to warm up your body before you begin exercising more vigorously. During that 5- to 10-minute warmup, rotate your arms, shoulders, and head gently to loosen your upper body. If you are cycling or swimming, do a few Arm Circles (page 53) and Shoulder Rolls (page 51) first, then ride or swim for a few minutes at a leisurely pace; in swimming, use a stroke that you enjoy most. If you are walking or riding a stationary bicycle, you will know that you are warmed up when you just begin to break a sweat.

Your Main Exercise Session

This is the time that really counts for fat burning! Adding no more than 5 minutes per week, work up to 30 minutes of continuous exercise at least four days per week, practicing the contemplation exercise each time. You should be walking (or riding, or swimming) hard enough so that you are breathing a little faster than usual, but not hard enough so you get winded.

Hints for walkers: Watch your posture: relax your shoulders, keep your chin down, and don't arch your lower back. Breathe through your nose at all times. Pumping your arms as you walk increases the aerobic benefit while building and toning muscles in the arms, shoulders, and upper and lower back. Bend elbows at a 90° angle, and loosely clench your fists. Move your arms straight forward and back, brushing the sides of your body. Though it may seem natural to let your arms cross toward the center of your body in the front, pumping straight forward and back requires more muscular control, is gentler on the shoulder joints, and helps to prevent low back pain.

Hints for swimmers: Use a variety of strokes: crawl/freestyle, breaststroke, sidestroke, backstroke. If you get winded, stop and tread water for a minute or two, or move to the side of the pool and practice some kicks (but try to maintain your contemplation exercise). Most authorities recommend continuing to move in some way during a recovery period rather than stopping completely. As your lung capacity improves, you'll be able to swim for longer periods. Note: there is some evidence that swimming is not as effective as dry-land exercise for losing body fat, because the water buoys you up and your muscles don't have to work as hard. Also, the cooling effect of the water means that your heart works less hard to do the same job. However, if you are new to exercise, swimming is a gentle, effective way to get into the exercise habit. You can also swim a few days per week, and walk or cycle other days. See the paragraph on "cross training," below.

Hints for cyclists: Your knees take less stress when you spin at a low gear (turn the cranks quickly and easily) instead of pushing a high gear (turn cranks slowly and with great effort). The combination of lower gear and fast cadence allows your muscles to work most efficiently. A long, steady ride trains your metabolism to burn fat more readily. If you are just starting out, take the time to choose a bicycle that fits correctly, and wear proper gear so that you remain comfortable. Find a location in your home where you can practice your contemplation exercise while riding, without becoming distracted by other family members, the television or radio, and so on.

Cross Training

Experienced athletes use cross training to increase their fitness and prevent injury. In cross training, you alternate two or, at the most, three forms of exercise during the week. Doing just one form of exercise trains only one set of muscles, while cross training works on different sets of muscles. For instance, cycling exercises the lower body primarily, while swimming focuses on the upper body. Swimming may not burn fat as fast as walking because it is not a weight-bearing exercise; however, walking is harder on the joints, especially the knees, and can be more strenuous for some people, especially if you are extremely sedentary. Doing a small amount of two forms of exercise prevents injury by varying the work that your joints and muscles are required to do. And of course, preventing injury means no lost time from daily exercise, which is an important component of any weight-management program. This technique also helps prevent boredom in your routine.

Wind Sprints (Interval Training)

A wind sprint is a short burst of higher intensity exercise in the middle of low-intensity exercise. For instance, after walking at your normal pace for 5-10 minutes, speed up to a much faster walk for 20-60 seconds, then slow back to your regular pace. Repeat every 5 to 10 minutes during your walking session. You can do the same while swimming or cycling. This short burst adds intensity to your exercise session without risking injury, and the brief extra work on your muscles means a more efficient fat-burning effect overall.

Cool Down

The cool-down period is as important as the warm-up. Walk, swim, or cycle at a slow pace for 5-10 minutes, then do a few stretches (on land) to lengthen the muscles that have contracted while you were exercising. If you don't stretch, your muscles will continue to contract and eventually start hurting due to the build-up of lactic acid. Here are some easy stretches that will work for either walking, swimming, or cycling:

Calf and Achilles' tendon stretches: (1) Stand facing a wall and rest your hands on the wall. Stand with back straight and abdominals in. Place right foot forward about six inches from the wall, and left foot back. Both heels remain flat on the floor, toes pointing forward. Ease your pelvis forward to feel the stretch in the main body of your left calf. Hold 10-15 seconds, then switch sides.

(2) Placing hands on the wall as before, stand with feet together about two feet away from the wall, toes forward and heels down. Keeping hips tucked in, gently bend knees until you feel the stretch in your lower calf and Achilles' tendon. Hold 10-15 seconds.

Toe Points and Ankle Circles: Holding on to a chair or bench for balance, straighten one leg in front of you and point your toes, then flex them. Repeat several times, then switch legs. Next, stretch one leg in front of you and rotate the ankle 5-10 times in each direction. Repeat with the other ankle.

Forward Bend: Stand with feet parallel, a few inches apart. Breathe in deeply, stretching your arms wide to the sides, then breathe out and bend forward, keeping your knees straight but not locked (if you have any lower back discomfort, you can bend your knees slightly). Let your upper body relax, especially your arms and head. Stay in the forward position for about 20 seconds, breathing normally. Then breathe in as you slowly straighten.

Heel back: Holding on to a chair or bench for balance with your left hand, bend your right knee and grasp the toes of your right foot behind you with your right hand. Pull the foot gently toward your body, stopping when you feel a pull in your thigh. Hold for about 20 seconds, breathing normally. Do this twice on each leg, alternating.

Shoulder stretch: Reach straight up with one hand as if trying to touch the ceiling. Now reach up behind your head with the other hand and pull the elbow across above your head slowly. Stop as soon as you feel a gentle pull in the shoulder, armpit, or back. Hold for a count of 20, breathing normally, then slowly release and relax. Do this twice on each side, alternating.

Chapter 8

Diet and Nutrition for Weight Management

The Yoga weight management diet is grounded in the idea of Nonviolence, the first and foremost of the ethical guidelines that are the basis of Yoga philosophy. When most people think about this ethic, they think of not harming others, but in Yoga practice your first duty is to not harm yourself. The strength of the partnership between your physical and spiritual bodies depends upon an attitude of help, not harm.

Achieving and maintaining normal weight is a good way to begin practicing Nonviolence toward yourself. We recommend doing this by balancing diet and physical activity, resulting in health and strength while losing weight safely. In this chapter, I will present a detailed outline of how to change your eating habits so that you can lose weight. If you are now of normal weight, these same suggestions, with just a little adjustment in calorie intake, can help you keep from gaining weight as you get older.

The Yogic approach to weight management is a lifestyle change that will help you all your life. The best quality of our Yoga program is that you will love doing it.

Counteracting Hunger and Inactivity

Most attempts at weight loss fail for one of three reasons: hunger, boredom, or inactivity. In Chapter 7, you learned some easy and enjoyable ways to increase your physical activity in order to help your body burn more calories. Now it's time to learn how to eat a well-balanced, healthy diet that will be so satisfying and varied that you won't feel so hungry and you won't be bored by your food choices.

Some fad diets seem to work great for a week or two, either by reducing calories in disguise by limiting foods to a few choices, such as the grapefruit diet, or by a diuretic (water loss) action, such as the low-carbohydrate diet. Only weight lost as body fat truly counts, so altering the water balance in your body has no long-term benefit. The currently popular low-carbohydrate, high-protein (which means high-fat) diets are good examples of diets that produce a short-term diuretic action. After an initial sharp reduction in weight associated with water loss, dieters quickly reach a plateau or even regain weight due to the typically high calorie content of the foods in this diet.

Despite what the popular magazines try to tell you, there is no magic pill or instant-success system for losing weight. There is no getting around the simple fact that to lose weight you must eat fewer calories than you burn up in physical activity. The easiest and healthiest way to burn more calories consistently is to exercise regularly and reduce your intake of the nonessential calories from the "calorie-dense" foods — those high in fat and/or sugar. This leaves you with plenty of nutritious foods to eat that not only build health, but also satisfy your hunger. I'll give you some specific examples later in the chapter.

It is essential to increase your activity level by following the routines outlined in this book; a nutritious diet cannot provide enough essential nutrients and still be low enough in calories for your body to burn fat. When you are inactive, your muscles start wasting away, and your percentage of body fat soars. Muscles burn many more calories than fat, so without exercising, you would have to restrict your calorie intake even more just to maintain a certain weight, much less lose extra pounds. It is also important to remember that metabolism naturally slows down with age, so a constant activity level is necessary to counteract these additional effects. The Yoga exercises presented in Chapter 3 help to maintain the most efficient metabolism; they are easy enough that they can be done every day, and many can be adapted for practice in a chair or even in bed, so the benefits can continue despite injury, illness, or age.

Why We Eat What We Eat

Try to become more aware of your ingrained associations with food. Food functions as much more than nourishment. As I discussed in Chapter 2, we often eat not because we are hungry but because of fear, or nervousness, or simply out of habit, such as what we used to eat as children. If you reached for a soft drink or a cookie for an after-school snack, you will tend to eat the same sort of snack as an adult. If your family commonly served dessert after a meal, you will expect something sweet after meals as an adult. There is nothing wrong with such habits if you are active enough and regulate your intake of calorie-dense foods enough to maintain normal weight.

One way to check your reactions to what and why you eat is with this variation of the wrist tape technique (see page 41 for complete instructions): Whenever you eat something, write "F" on the tape if you are eating because your body needs fuel, "B" if you are eating because you are bored, or "S" if you are stressed. At the end of the week, add up the three categories to show you how your mood affects how you eat. Food only makes you fat when it is used to make yourself feel better, to entertain yourself, or to get rid of tension, as opposed to eating simply to nourish your body.

Strange Medical Notes – I

Chewing gum can help you lose weight! Researchers measured energy expenditure in volunteers before and after chewing gum for 12 minutes at a steady rate (100 chews per minute, using a metronome), and found an increase in calorie-burning after the gum-chewing session. They figured that gum chewing could help you lose about 11 pounds per year. Unfortunately, to achieve this weight loss, you'd have to chew at the prescribed pace during every waking hour of every day!

Essential Nutrients

The key concept is essentiality: Learn what nutrients are required for health and learn how to create a diet that contains them in concentrated form, without adding unnecessary calories from nonessential fats and sugars. The best weight management diet simply reduces or eliminates the nonessential.

Protein

The average American diet supplies about twice as much as is needed, usually accompanied by very nonessential saturated fat. Protein is required for building and repairing tissue, and for hormone production. Protein seems to play the primary role in the brain in reducing the hunger sensation, so if your weight management diet is sufficient in protein, it may help reduce cravings and hunger pangs.

On an extremely low-calorie diet, the body may "panic," believing that it is starving. It then sets the body's metabolic rate lower in order to conserve energy, which prevents weight loss. To avoid this, be sure that protein is adequate in your weight management diet. Protein should constitute about 15% of your caloric intake. If you follow the suggested diet plan in this chapter and obtain all the required servings of protein each day, you will be getting adequate protein.

Protein sources

The best low-fat protein sources are fat-free dairy products (milk, yogurt, and cottage cheese); "fake" meats made from soy products; and pure protein pills (amino acid tablets). Other sources of protein, such as meats; peas, beans, and lentils; and tofu, are somewhat higher in protein but also higher in fat. Many whole grains contain a small amount of protein as well. If you eat meat, buy it as lean as possible.

Pure protein tablets provide as much as 1.9 grams of high-grade natural dairy protein per tablet. Since the tablets are pure protein, this source is the most efficient at delivering the maximum amount of protein for the lowest number of calories. Plus, they are easily portable, so you can maintain your weight management diet in restaurants and at work or play. When using a pure source such as this, it is important to supplement your diet with iron and zinc as well as other vitamins and minerals that naturally accompany protein foods. There is a fuller discussion of vitamin/mineral supplementation at the end of this chapter.

Carbohydrates

Carbohydrates are the best source of calories to fuel your muscles and brain. If your body has to burn protein or fat, toxic by-products are formed. For this reason, I do not recommend low-carbohydrate diets. Instead, I recommend getting about 55% of daily calories from carbohydrate foods such as vegetables, peas and beans, fruits, bread, pasta, and cereal.

Fiber

Here is another good reason to concentrate on carbohydrates: High-carbohydrate foods such as fruits, vegetables, and whole grains are also usually high in fiber. High-fiber diets contribute to long-term cardiovascular health by lowering insulin levels. A high intake of fiber in the diet is also associated with lower weight. Alternatively, those whose diets are low in fiber, and therefore eat more meat and dairy products, are more likely to be overweight.

Nonessential, Calorie-Dense Foods

Animal fats such as butter, lard, and meat fat are saturated and contribute to heart disease and some cancers. Vegetable fats such as grain, seed, and nut oils tend to be less saturated and less harmful, but all have the same high calorie content and are equally nonessential. There is an important exception: the essential fatty acids that are needed primarily for hormone production. However, only one teaspoon or so of vegetable oil daily (approximately 30 calories worth) amply supplies this requirement. Though the vast majority of dietary fats are nonessential to health, we crave them because they help create a satiated feeling. Note: The diet suggestions in this book are intended only for adults; children under 16 need a greater percentage of dietary fat to facilitate the growth process, although establishing healthy eating habits early will help prevent weight gain as an adult. Consult a registered dietician for help in preventing or treating overweight in children.

Here is where the greatest cuts in calorie consumption can be made in your diet. The type of fat you should cut back on most is the saturated variety from meats, butterfat (any dairy products except fat-free) and the vegetable fats found in coconut and palm oils (these are added to a great many processed foods). Foods that usually contain the most saturated fat are meats, butter, ice cream, nondairy creamers, and baked goods. Fried foods invariably absorb some of the cooking fat, adding nonessential calories, and this includes potato and corn chips.

Vegetarianism

Throughout this chapter I will be emphasizing a healthy, low-fat vegetarian diet. That is what I have followed for over 45 years, and it is the traditional diet for serious Yoga students, because it is nonviolent. You do not have to be a vegetarian to practice Yoga. However, just in terms of volume, there is no doubt that a healthy vegetarian weight-loss diet gives you more to eat than a diet that includes meat, because meat products are so calorie-dense.

How to Create a Balanced Diet

A balanced diet means several things, all required for health and successful weight management. If you are already overweight, your energy intake (calories) has exceeded your energy expenditure (physical activity) for a period of time sufficient to add on the extra pounds. Most people in this situation try to lose weight by excluding most foods, no matter how important for good health, and eating a very unbalanced diet relying on a few favored items. A typical lunch might be a plain bagel and a salad, with black coffee. This type of weight loss diet deprives the body of essential nutrients, especially protein. Not only does this type of diet result in the body's immediate alarm of impending starvation, which, as I mentioned earlier, changes the way energy is processed, it also affects growth, hormones, and healing. Not to mention the fact that it soon becomes so boring and distasteful that you can't stand to keep it up, so in the long run it does not work.

Happy Changes

I would advise a very slow approach to any change in your eating habits. This will enable you to succeed in small ways every day. Gradually, after a week or so, you will easily be able to set your daily intake goal and happily stay with it. If you suddenly impose rigid requirements on yourself, both the inner and outer body will react in upset.

Begin with replacing three items that are high-calorie intake with low-calorie, chewable replacements. Make it easy on yourself. For instance, if you want two cookies for dessert, eat one and then eat a carrot or a piece of an apple to replace what you have lost. Realize carefully what you have done and cajole both bodies with the inner conversation that you have given your physical body what it wants and that you are also proud and appreciative of the emotional support that was provided from the inner body.

The best way to lose unwanted pounds is to change your lifestyle to a more healthy balance of "energy in," through food, and "energy out," through activity. Remember that it may take as long to return to a normal weight as it took to gain it in the first place. Don't be discouraged; instead of thinking "I am dieting," think: "I am eating today the way I want to be eating next year and the year after." Go for the long term, not the short term, and develop some plan for yourself that you love.

If your weight is now in the normal range, you can prevent becoming overweight (and improve your health overall) by following these suggestions:

• Eat a variety of foods

• Match your food intake with your level of physical activity

• Choose a diet with plenty of grain products, vegetables, and fruits

• Choose a diet low in fat, saturated fat, and cholesterol

• Eat only moderate amounts of sugar, salt, and processed foods with added sodium

• Moderate your intake of alcohol

• Remember, when choosing foods, that 1 gram of fat = 9 calories, while 1 gram of carbohydrate or protein = only 4 calories, less than half as much.

Calories eaten earlier in the day are more likely to be burned up in physical activity than the same calories eaten at night before bed. Also, you are more likely to eat more calories per day if you starve during the day and "eat normally" at night. Most people who try to diet this way become so hungry by the end of the day that "normal" quickly becomes "too much." This is not a nonviolent approach, because your physical body becomes depleted and fatigued during the day, and your emotional body suffers from neglect of its needs as well. There is an old adage that says, "Eat breakfast like a king, lunch like a prince, and supper like a pauper." An easy way to think about what to eat at night is to try to eat only nonfat, nonsugary foods after 6 PM.

Unfortunately, the current trend in our society seems to be diverging ever farther from healthy eating habits as we become ever more inactive, or exercise in place of eating a meal. For instance, many like to start the day with a morning jog or other exercise session, but then have no time to eat a decent breakfast, grabbing a high-fat, fast-food sandwich or pastry to eat while driving to work or at their desk.

A recent National Public Radio story reported that breakfast is now the meal most likely to be skipped; substantially less than half of Americans eat breakfast every day. One of the many reasons cited was increased commuting times as traffic congestion continues to increase and the suburbs to expand. No mention is made of the fractured relationships that come from the "I don't have time for breakfast" attitude.

Weight Loss Tip

Eat meals sitting down, and pace your eating, because before you feel full enough to quit eating, food has to enter your bloodstream and send the right signals to your brain to tell you that you have had enough — and this takes at least 20 minutes. Eat slowly and enjoy your meal. It is often a good idea to start with a low-calorie salad or a broth-type soup to make the meal last longer and fill you up sooner.

The ideal breakfast includes low-fat, high-fiber carbohydrate foods such as low-sugar cereal with fat-free milk, or perhaps dry whole wheat toast and soft-boiled or poached eggs. Hot cereal, especially oatmeal, is also a great alternative. You also do not have to stick to traditional "breakfast" foods. Here are some examples of nutritious, low-calorie breakfast meals that can be prepared and eaten in a hurry:

• Shake made by blending 1 cup fat-free milk, 1 banana, 3 or 4 strawberries or handful of blueberries (for extra satisfaction, add a tablespoon of nutritional [not baking] yeast, which may be found in health food stores).

• Whole-grain bagel sandwich with lettuce, mustard, and fat-free, meat-alternative Canadian bacon; fat-free cottage cheese on the side.

• Hard-boiled egg; whole-grain toast with small amount of no-added-sugar preserves.

The Yoga Weight Management Diet

We are basing our suggestions for a weight-loss diet on the USDA food guide pyramid, which suggests how to build your daily diet in terms of servings of different food groups. If you are on a weight-gain-prevention diet, you eat more servings and can choose higher calorie foods from each group; if you are trying to lose weight, you eat fewer servings and choose lower calorie foods. Before setting out the specific diet plan, I want to tell you more about the Food Guide Pyramid and offer some general suggestions about reducing fat and sugar in your diet.

The Food Guide Pyramid

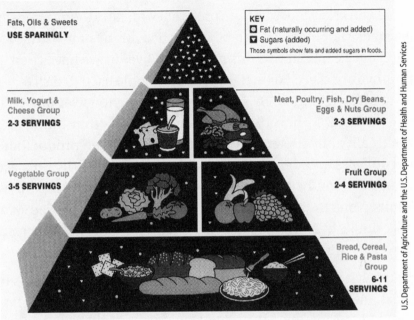

Starting from the lowest, widest level, the food guide pyramid emphasizes carbohydrates, allowing the greatest number of servings for these healthy fuel foods:

Grains:
Bread, cereal, rice, and pasta: 6 - 11 servings

Fruits and vegetables:
Vegetables: 3 - 5 servings

Fruits: 2 - 4 servings

Protein:
Dairy: 2 - 3 servings

Meat, poultry, fish,
dry beans, eggs, & nuts: 2 - 3 servings

Fats, oils, and sweets:
No requirement. Use sparingly.

How to Reduce Fats

Did you know that our taste preference for fatty foods is mostly learned? That means it can be unlearned. Many of my students and I have experienced this in our own lives as we have tried to improve our diets. For instance, many people used to dislike the taste of fat-free milk. By gradually switching to lower fat products — first 2%, then 1%, and finally fat-free — they found that eventually they preferred the taste of the fat-free product and did not miss the added fat. It works the same with butter on toast, sour cream on baked potatoes, and other culturally ingrained habits. Note: Recently some milk producers have improved skim milk simply by adding fat-free milk solids, resulting in better taste as well as more protein and calcium.

I think it is heartening to find out that when we take pains to break these fat habits, we find that we prefer the taste and texture of foods without the added fat. Take a "fat vacation" for a month, and then see what fats you really cannot live without. Add the "must haves" back as sparingly as possible. For instance, if butter is on your list, eat it on Sunday only. If you are like most, you can enjoy food and eating just as much with markedly less fat than you are used to! Here's how to reduce fats in the major food groups of the pyramid:

First, let's talk about grains. How can we make sure this carbohydrate foundation to our diet is not too high in fat? First, try taking the "no-spread pledge"! This means eating breads and toast without spreading on the butter or margarine. When eating breakfast in a restaurant, remember to ask for "dry whole wheat toast, please." If at first you can't face toast with no spread at all, try a small amount of no-added-sugar preserves or fat-free cream cheese. It is easy to find a cereal without added sugar, and simply by switching to fat-free milk, you are well on the way toward a really low-fat, low-calorie breakfast.

No-Fat Foolery

Remember that fat-free does not mean calorie-free! Many packaged items increase sugars and other calorie-dense ingredients in order to compensate for the reduced fat in their product. Read labels, and try to avoid eating packaged foods as much as possible. Especially enjoy the labels on such products as chocolate syrup and even apples, which say "as always, fat-free"!

Do you always put gravy or butter on rice? Try serving rice as many Asians do, as a layer under low-fat vegetables or beans, peas, or lentils. Pasta dishes can be low-fat or high-fat items depending on the sauce. Do you know that Italian-style canned tomato pasta sauces vary from 0% to at least 50% of calories from fat? Many of the fat-free varieties are quite tasty. Remember, if it is a creamy pasta sauce, it probably is high fat, and saturated to boot. If you really prefer the taste of a creamy sauce, sauté vegetables in a small amount of oil (use a canola oil pan spray) and stir fat-free yogurt into the pan after taking it off the heat for a low-fat creamy pasta topping. You can also try the more traditional approach of tossing the hot pasta and the sautéed vegetables with skim-milk ricotta cheese.

Unfortunately, there is no easy way to reduce the fat in cakes, cookies, and muffins unless you bake them yourself. If you do, you can substitute nonfat yogurt or applesauce for some or all of the butter or oil in the recipe. If high-fat foods such as pie crusts, croissants, and doughnuts are on your list of "must-haves," you'll have to limit them to once a week or less in order to truly benefit from a low-fat diet. There are a few things you can do to somewhat reduce the fat in these foods; for instance, if pie is a favorite food, eat one-crust pies instead of double-crust.

How about vegetables? Frying vegetables of any kind moves them from the highly recommended list all the way to the "use sparingly" list. The same for butter or cheese sauces for vegetables. Flavor your veggies with fresh herbs, lemon juice, and a little salt and pepper, or cook them with onions and garlic. Sauté them quickly in a nonstick pan, with perhaps a quick blast from a canola oil pan spray. Even the large portabello mushroom can be pan grilled this way! If a butter sauce is on your list of "must haves," try one of the instant natural butter flavor mixes.

Fruits are perhaps the best food for a weight management diet because they are naturally full of carbohydrates, have a sweet taste, and are usually eaten with no added fat. The only fatty fruit habit that could be a problem is peanut butter on bananas.

At the dairy level, milk and yogurt are readily available in a range of fat content from 0 to 4%, and some brands of cottage, ricotta, and even Swiss, cheddar, and mozzarella cheeses are available in fat-free form. We were delighted to discover that even half-and-half has a new fat-free form, although it still contains over 50% more calories than fortified skim milk.

Now we come to a very difficult group — one that is often loaded with fat built right into the foods themselves. Meat, poultry, and fish dishes usually contain high amounts of saturated fat unless special efforts are made to purchase and prepare low-fat versions of typical recipes. Dried beans are traditionally cooked with added fat, egg yolks are high in cholesterol, which is a form of fat, and nuts are so high in fat they are even a good commercial source of oil. Perhaps peas and lentils are not so often loaded up with added fats as the other members of the group, but even here caution is needed. Split pea soup traditionally is prepared with added meat fat, and Indian methods of cooking the various legumes (dal) usually call for flavoring with clarified butter (ghee). In order to limit nonessential fat in this group, choose well-trimmed, low-fat meat, skinless poultry, grilled skinless fish, poached or boiled eggs (no more than 3 - 4 per week unless you use one of the many liquid fat-free egg substitutes), nontraditional fat-free preparations of peas, beans, and lentils, and very limited amounts of nuts.

Soy products are increasingly in evidence in major supermarkets, and their low-fat or nonfat varieties are an excellent source of protein. Certainly the "fake meat" wieners, burgers, Canadian bacon, and deli slices are healthier for you than the meats they mimic. Even if you are not a vegetarian, you will benefit from adding some of these foods to your diet; eating a "veggie" hot dog or slice of bacon as a snack is a great comfort for hunger pangs. Most people are familiar with soybean curd (tofu), a staple food of Asia; it is a bland cakelike high-protein food that can be barbecued, scrambled, sautéed with vegetables, boiled, or baked. When processed with calcium, as it usually is, tofu is a great source of this essential mineral as well as protein. My local supermarket now carries tempeh, a fermented soy cake that has more texture and flavor than tofu and is higher in protein. For cooking suggestions, consult any vegetarian cookbook (see Resources).

Strange Medical Notes – II

Green tea may help with weight loss, say researchers. They gave volunteers three daily doses of green tea extract or a comparable amount of caffeine. They found a small but significant increase in energy expenditure in people receiving the green tea extract. Unlike stimulant-containing diet drugs, the green tea did not increase heart rate, and so is probably not a danger to overweight people with high blood pressure or heart disease.

Eating in Restaurants

Most restaurants, especially the fast-food establishments, seem to specialize in adding fat to foods; that's what they do best! Serving sizes have also grown and grown; in some major chains the amount of food on your plate can easily contain a whole day's requirements of calories. I remember well when a dietician, noting a major food chain's newest big burger, remarked that of course it wasn't too high in fat: just buy one on Monday, cut it into five pieces and eat a piece every day! Fried foods top the list of favorite restaurant foods. If it's fried, it's high in fat, and if it's batter-fried it's doubly high. That also goes for refried items, cheese sauces, melted cheese, or cream sauce. Almost any whitish dipping sauce is code for mayonnaise, which means vegetable oil. Always ask for salad dressing on the side, and use as little as you can. You may discover you actually like and prefer the unadorned taste of vegetables.

When you order breakfast toast, forget about the yellow-colored fat carefully brushed from crust to crust; ask for dry toast and add your own butter or margarine or preserves, sparingly.

Sometimes dry whole wheat toast and poached eggs are the only low-fat choices available; even oatmeal is a little unusual these days. Granola is a blatant contradiction: widely associated with health, it is often high in both added fat and sugar. Pancakes can be a good choice, especially if you can find some with fiber, such as buckwheat, and limit the amount of added fat (butter, margarine) and sugar (syrup, jelly) you add.

Lunch can include salads, bread, and baked potatoes at most establishments. Deli sandwiches can be improved by replacing mayonnaise with mustard, lettuce, and tomato, using whole-grain bread products, and removing at least half the cheese or meat filling. Chinese food can be a good alternative if you select stir-fried vegetable and bean curd dishes with plain rice. Mexican food should probably be saved for rare special occasions; fried and refried foods are the order of the day, and even avocados are 93% calories from fat. Try to order plain flour tortillas, rice, beans (not refried!) and remove extra cheese from items such as tostados, tacos, burritos, and enchiladas.

Feeding Both Your Bodies

If you are faced with a high-fat burrito, taco, or other food, divide it into three parts. Eat one for your emotional body, one for your physical body, then fantasize stuffing the other part into your unwilling hips and waist as they protest. If your emotional body fights for more, mark your wrist tape (see page 41) and figure out how to make up the loss to it. This will show you if you are constantly denying your inner emotional body and help you to notice when it rebels. This technique will work with any high-fat or high-sugar foods — you can even divide up all your meals this way just for fun.

How To Reduce Added Sugars

There is nothing intrinsically unhealthy about sugar, but it is a nonessential food, and it adds calories without adding nourishment, so sweets should be eaten only sparingly. Here are some ways to reduce sugar in the other food groups:

Grain products can very easily become loaded with added sugar. Breakfast cereals out of the box can seem like candy; toast is often slathered with jam or jelly; and cakes, cookies, and muffins all have a great deal of added sugar, unless you make them yourself. Try cutting the amount of sugar in half; you'll be surprised at how sweet the finished product is. Read the labels on processed foods, and be alert for the total amount of sugar in a product. For instance, in order to avoid having sugar at the top of their list of ingredients, some cereal manufacturers disguise the total amount by separately listing many different kinds of sugar such as honey, corn syrup, maple syrup, glucose, and fructose.

Vegetables are not likely to be prepared with added sugar. Fruits, on the other hand, are often candied, packed in syrup, or made into jams, jellies, or preserves. If you buy canned fruit, choose varieties packed in their own juice, with no added sugar. Choose fruit-only preserves, and buy fruit juices that are 100% juice.

In the dairy group, sweetened, fruit-filled yogurt is the only product likely to contain added sugar, unless you are still a kid at heart and drink chocolate milk or are addicted to ice cream! Even then, there are many low-fat and even some fat-free and sugar-free varieties to try, such as fat-free, sugar-free frozen yogurt and ice milk.

America's Sugar Overload

Added sweeteners account for about 16% of calories in most American diets — almost double the recommended amount. Added sweeteners are found most often in soft drinks, and consumption of soft drinks is steadily increasing. Besides adding unwanted calories, these drinks replace more nutritious food; for instance, teenage girls and young women need the calcium in milk to help prevent osteoporosis (brittle bones). If you are trying to lose weight, soft drinks — even the "sugar-free" varieties — won't help. Better choices are water, nonfat milk, or sparkling water flavored with lemon or a small amount of pure fruit juice.

The protein group is unlikely to contain added sugar except for unusual items such as processed meats, which you would be avoiding anyway because of the high fat content, not to mention added chemicals. I try to avoid artificial colors and flavors at all times, because I want to eat food, not chemicals.

How Many Calories Do I Need?

Now we come to the diet plan itself. The type of plan that you select depends mainly upon your activity level; the more active you are, the more calories you can eat and still lose weight.

STEP 1: Determine your usual activity level by identifying the category that BEST describes your TYPICAL day:

Low Activity Level — slowly paced or seated activities such as work seated at a desk, riding in a car or other vehicle, watching television, walking, shopping, bowling, fishing, golf, housework, standing work, light gardening (weeding, grass cutting, pruning, etc.).

Moderate Activity Level — briskly paced activities, such as at least one hour daily (not necessarily consecutive) brisk walking, swimming, dancing, or recreational sport or calisthenics, moderate gardening (cultivating, shoveling, raking, etc.).

High Activity Level — minimum of two hours daily (not necessarily consecutive) of fast-paced activities such as heavy manual labor, jogging/running, competitive sports.

STEP 2: Using one of the following charts, determine how many calories you require to keep your weight stable at your typical activity level.

Find your current weight in the left column and your activity level in the top row on one of the charts below. Where the two intersect is your calorie requirement to maintain that weight.

It is clear that men and women have very different needs. It is also clear that activity makes a big difference — a 50% difference!

Women's Calorie Requirements

Weight in Pounds	Activity Level		
	Low	Moderate	High
100	1224	1428	1836
110	1262	1473	1894
120	1301	1518	1951
130	1339	1562	2009
140	1378	1607	2066
150 (152 is average)	1416	1652	2124
160	1454	1697	2182
170	1493	1742	2239
180	1531	1786	2297
190	1570	1831	2354
200	1608	1876	2412

STEP 3: Determine if you want to lose weight or simply prevent becoming overweight.

To do this, refer back to your Body Mass Index (BMI), described in Chapter 1. A BMI less than 25 is most desirable and means that all you have to do is maintain your present weight; a BMI between 25 and 30 should encourage you to reduce your weight. If your BMI is higher than 30 you should check with your doctor for supervised weight reduction.

Men's Calorie Requirements

Weight in Pounds	Activity Level		
	Low	Moderate	High
150	1890	2205	2835
160	1944	2268	2916
170	1998	2331	2997
180 (average)	2052	2394	3078
190	2106	2457	3159
200	2160	2520	3240
210	2214	2583	3321
220	2268	2646	3402
230	2322	2709	3483
240	2376	2772	3564
250	2430	2835	3645

STEP 4: Refer to the Diet Plan Table on page 165.

If your BMI falls within the acceptable range, find your present weight calorie range across the top and then read down to determine the servings and types of foods that will help you maintain your weight. Example: If you are a man who is moderately active and wishes to maintain a 180-pound stable weight, you need 2394 calories per day. In the Diet Plan Table, you would choose the plan in column F.

If you need to lose some weight to reduce your BMI, you need to reduce your stable weight calories. Keep in mind that to lose one pound per week, you need a 500-calorie deficit every day. Do not reduce calories alone! Reduce some calories and increase activity instead. The result is the same as far as weight loss is concerned, but by increasing activity, your future weight will be lower. So, after finding your current weight on the table above, subtract 500 calories. On the Diet Plan Table, find the reduced calorie level across the top and then read down to determine the servings and types of foods for you.

Example: If you are a woman who has a low activity level and now weighs 160 pounds, your maintenance calorie level is 1454 calories. To lose a pound a week through diet restriction alone, you would have to choose a diet plan that allows 500 calories fewer, or only 954 calories. We do not recommend eating fewer than 1200 calories per day without strict physician supervision (see Chapter 1 for more about safe calorie goals); therefore, if you wish to lose one pound per week you will need to boost your activity level so that you can lose weight on 1200 calories according to the diet plan in column A. Do not restrict calories below 1200!

Earlier, I talked about the fact that it may take as much time to lose unwanted weight as it took to put the weight on in the first place. If you think back, you probably did not gain the unwanted weight in a short period of time. Most people who are not watching their diet may gain 10-15 pounds per year. Thus, if you truly change your eating habits so that you can maintain a healthy, gradual weight-loss diet, you may lose at that same slow-but-steady rate.

Remember that physical activity increases your muscle mass and metabolic rate, which helps to keep weight off for the long term. For each 30 minutes of brisk activity each day, you can add back 135 calories (180 for men) in the Diet Plan Table. Additional exercise is the best solution also for smaller people who hit the 1200-calorie limit, because they can increase weight loss goals without reducing calories to dangerous levels.

What Is a Serving?

In the Diet Plan Table above, notice that some serving amounts are labeled "low" and the rest are labeled "other." Because calorie counts for different foods vary widely, we suggest that you choose your foods mostly from the lower calorie groups; foods in the "other" category tend to be higher in calories. Here are some examples from each group (see Resources for a list of books and Internet sites to use to find your own calorie counts):

Grains:

Low-calorie (avg. 70 cal./serv.)	Other (avg. 100 cal.)
Bow-tie pasta (1/2 c)	Elbow macaroni (1/2 c)
Weight Watchers oat bran bread (1 slice)	Raisin bread (1 slice)
Total Multigrain cornflakes (1 c)	Cheerios (1 c)
Cooked cereal (1/2 c)	White short- grain rice (1 c)

Diet Plan Table

	A	B	C	D	E	F
Calories	1200-1400	1400-1600	1600-1800	1800-2000	2000-2200	2200-2400
Grains	6 low	3 low, 3 other	2 low, 4 other	9 low	5 low, 4 other	3 low, 6 other
Vegetables	3 low	2 low, 1 other	2 low, 2 other	5 low	3 low, 2 other	2 low, 3 other
Fruits	2 low	1 low, 1 other	2 other	4 low	2 low, 2 other	4 other
Dairy	2 low	2 low	2 low	3 low	3 low	3 low
Protein	3 low	3 low	2 other	2 other	3 other	6 low, or 3/3
Fats, Sugars	none*	sparing				

*This diet plan includes 100 calories per day for a snack or some other "free food" of your choice.

Vegetables (1/2 c servings unless otherwise noted):

Low calorie (avg. 17 cal.)	Other (avg. 64 cal.)
Asparagus	Winter squash
Broccoli	Corn
Beans, green	Peas
Cauliflower	Tomato sauce (canned)
Zucchini	Potato w/skin (1 med)

Fruits:

Low calorie (avg. 40 cal.)	Other (avg. 102 cal.)
Apple (1 med)	Apricots, dried (10 halves)
Blueberries (1/2 c)	Pear (1 med)
Grapes (10)	Banana (1 med)
Honeydew melon (1/8 melon)	Raisins (1/4 c)

Dairy:

Low calorie (avg. 90 cal.)	Other (avg. 180 cal.)
Skim milk (1 c)	Whole milk (1 c)
Plain yogurt (1 c)	Fruited nonfat yogurt (1 c)
2% cottage cheese (1/2 c)	Parmesan cheese (2 oz)
Light Swiss cheese (1 oz)	Cheddar cheese (1 oz)

Protein:

Low calorie (avg. 113 cal.)	Other (avg. 189 cal.)
Tofu, firm (3 oz)	Tempeh (4 oz)
Yves veg. weiner (1)	Chicken broiled (3 oz)
Yves Canadian bacon (4 slices)	Hamburger broiled (3 oz)
Dried beans (1/2 c cooked)	Beef, lean roasted (3 oz)

How To Cheat!

First, let's not call it cheating; let's call it being kind to both your bodies! If you find yourself really hungry, don't give up. Eat an extra grain serving along with a small serving of a protein-rich food — example: a piece of good bread with a glass of fat-free milk. Avoid telling yourself "I've failed, I've blown it, there's no point in continuing," because you have not failed. You have begun a new relationship with your emotional body in a new awareness of its need to be happy. Second, avoid eating fatty foods; even in small portions they won't be as satisfying as a larger portion of carbohydrate and protein. Remember, carbohydrate foods are much less likely to be stored as body fat than the same calories from fatty foods.

Sample Menus

Following are sample menus for two of the six diet plans shown in the Diet Plan Table. The calorie count for each menu skews toward the lower end of the range: for example, the sample menu for column A totals about 1200 calories, even though the range is from 1200 to 1400 calories. You can easily adjust your calorie level upward by substituting an "other" choice for a low-calorie choice, or by adding 100 calories or so in a favorite snack. (See Resources for some excellent books and Internet sources that can help you create your own menus.)

Sample menu for column "A" (1200-1400 calories)

Breakfast

1c milk (fortified skim)	110	1 dairy
1c Product 19 cereal	100	1 grain
1/2 small banana	60	1 fruit
1/2 bagel	80	1 grain
	———	
	350	

Lunch

1/2 c tomato soup	90	1 veg
2 slices Weight Watcher's Oat bran bread	80	2 grain
4 slices Yves Veggie Pepperoni	90	1 protein
lettuce/tomato	25	1 veg
mustard	--	--
1/2 c melon	30	1 fruit
	———	
	315	

Snack

1 c yogurt — plain or artificially sweetened, nonfat	90	1 dairy

Dinner

Omelet made with 2 egg substitutes and 1/2 c veggies and 1 slice veg. Can. bacon	182	2 protein, 1 veg
1 tsp butter	45	1 fat
1 c mixed green salad	25	1 veg
2 Tbs fat free dressing	45	
1 slice whole-wheat toast	86	1 grain
1 tsp low-sugar spread	25	
	408	

Snack

2 rice cakes	80	1 grain

1243 Total Calories

Sample menu for Column "B" (1400-1600 calories)

Breakfast

Breakfast burrito	230	1 protein, 1 grain
Milk, 1 c	110	1 dairy
Papaya, 1/2 med	60	1 fruit
	400	

Lunch

Veggie Burger, Morningstar Farms	70	1 protein
Bun	60	2 grain
Kraft fat-free Swiss, 1 slice	30	1 dairy
Red onion, tomatoes	29	1 veg
Mixed green salad	19	1 veg
Fat-free dressing	33	
Peach	37	1 fruit
	——	
	278	

Snacks

Snack Wells fat free crackers (5)	60	1 grain
Carrot sticks and fat-free Vegetable dip	109	1 veg
	——	
	169	

Dinner

Ziti (1 c) with zucchini 1/2 c	232	2 grain, 1 veg
1 TB Parmesan ch	100	
Fruit salad, 1 c	101	2 fruit

1 c V-8 Juice	56	1 veg
Whole wheat roll	74	1 grain
	——	
	563	
	—————	

1410 Total Calories

Supplementing Your Diet

Food First!

Vitamins and minerals cannot replace food. Foods have hundreds of undiscovered chemicals that may be important to health; vitamin and mineral supplements have only a handful. It is best to eat a wide variety of foods and to avoid chemical excesses and imbalances. Don't be one of the 9 out of 10 Americans who do not regularly eat the recommended number of daily servings of fruits and vegetables! The best strategy for optimal health and reducing your risk of chronic disease is to obtain adequate nutrients from a wide variety of foods.

Having said that, there are some instances in which supplementation may be a wise course. If you are severely restricting calories in order to lose weight, vitamins and minerals may well be undersupplied. Even a well-balanced diet can be lacking in adequate amounts if you restrict quantity and portion size. Generally, if you tend to skip meals, diet often, or eat meals high in sugar and fat, supplements are a reasonable course.

Who Should Supplement?

Besides those on a restricted-calorie diet, there are other groups of people who would probably benefit from supplementation. Older people and teenagers often have irregular eating habits and do not eat a well-balanced diet. Many older adults are at least mildly overweight and often restrict choices and amounts of food even further. Depression, lack of appetite, loss of taste and smell, and denture problems can all contribute to an older person not eating well. Absorption of vitamins can be impaired in older people. Teens are often self-conscious about their weight and may restrict food intake without knowing how to do it wisely. Older women often need extra vitamin D and calcium for protection from osteoporosis, and teens often do not get enough calcium to grow strong bones. Supplements can help to make up for these shortages.

Women have special needs throughout life, starting with calcium and vitamin D to prevent osteoporosis, as mentioned above. Women of child-bearing years usually do not get enough folic acid, which reduces neurological birth defects. Doctors usually prescribe vitamin and mineral supplements for pregnant and lactating women, whose requirements are higher during this time.

Vegans (vegetarians who eat absolutely no animal products, including dairy and eggs) are unlikely to get adequate amounts of vitamins B-2 and B-12, or calcium, iron, and zinc, and should consider supplementation.

Best Food Sources — Vitamins

A simple rule of thumb: grains for B-complex, fruits and vegetables for vitamins A, C, and E. Citrus, bananas, cantaloupe, and dried fruits are all excellent; the vegetables with the highest vitamin content are always the most colorful ones! Dark green leafy vegetables such as spinach, colorful peppers, and all the members of the cabbage family such as broccoli, cauliflower, brussels sprouts, and cabbage itself, along with carrots and winter squash, are all excellent sources.

All B-complex vitamins are included in whole grain products (except for B-12, which is found in milk, eggs, and meat). Eggs also supply most of the other B-complex vitamins, as do many fruits, vegetables, and meat. Vitamin D is added to milk and is formed on the skin by sunlight. Everyone should take a supplement with 400 mcg of folic acid.

Best Food Sources — Minerals

Iron is found in high amounts in beef and pork and in moderate amounts in prunes, apricots, spinach, beans, tofu, blackstrap molasses, nutritional yeast, and wheat germ. However, all sources are dwarfed by the iron content of fortified cereals. For example, Total brand cereal contains 18 mg of iron, which is 100% of the recommended daily intake. Younger people, especially premenopausal women, need the 18 mg DV (daily value) of iron, but older men and women should be fine with 0 to 10 mg daily.

Zinc is much more difficult to obtain, with only beef, pork, and shellfish being good sources. Wheat germ, garbanzo beans, and lentils are the best of the rest, but in order to get the recommended 15 mg, you would need to eat nearly 1¹/₂ cups of wheat germ, for instance. A mineral supplement supplying the recommended amount of zinc seems to make good sense.

Calcium is highest in dairy foods: milk, yogurt, and cheese. Other good sources include tofu (if processed with calcium sulfate) and dark green leafy vegetables (spinach, turnip greens, kale, etc.). Unless you commit to eating at least four servings per day of high-calcium dairy foods (1 serving = 1 cup milk, 1 cup yogurt, 1 oz hard cheese), a calcium supplement should be used to replace the missing calcium. Calcium supplements should total 900 – 1,000 mg per day (three 300-mg tablets or two 500-mg tablets for older people).

Trace minerals are difficult to evaluate and should be sufficient in the diet provided unrefined foods such as whole grains and fresh fruits and vegetables provide the majority of calories. The single exception is selenium. Add 200 mcg selenium to your supplement list for protection from prostate, lung, and colon cancers.

How to Supplement

Here are three ways to be sure you are getting an adequate amount of essential vitamins and minerals:

1. The best choice is to eat moderate amounts of a wide variety of foods prepared in such a way as to preserve the naturally occurring vitamins and minerals. The most nutritious foods suitable for a weight management diet are fat-free dairy products; deeply colored fruits and vegetables such as carrots, spinach, apricots, mangos, winter squash, and tomatoes; whole-grain bread and cereal products; and good protein sources such as

soy-based meat substitutes, dried beans and peas, and, if you eat meat, lean cuts of meat, poultry, and fish. If some of the choices mentioned here don't sound appetizing to you, do some research and find some nutritious alternatives that you do like. It's important to eat food that you enjoy.

2. If you are unable or unlikely to follow option #1, consider taking a complete multivitamin/multimineral supplement daily. Look for those that provide at least 100% of the daily value for A, B-1, B-2, niacin, B-6, B-12, C, D, E, and folic acid. Limit beta carotene to no more than 15,000 IU, iron to 18 mg, phosphorous to 500 mg, and B-6 to 200 mg. The supplement should also provide at least 25 mcg of vitamin K, 120 mcg of chromium, 100 mg magnesium, 2 mg copper, and 15 mg zinc. Iron requirements vary with gender and age: Women under 50 need 8 to 18 mg of iron, men under 50 need under 10 mg, and men and women over 50 need no more than 10 mg iron. Everyone over 50 needs at least 24 mcg of B-12, because of generally poor absorption in older bodies.

A comprehensive multivitamin/mineral is a simple and relatively inexpensive choice. You do not need to spend a lot of money on a supplement; the cheapest brands are often as well-balanced and effective as the more expensive brands. I do not care for artificial coloring myself, so I choose uncolored brands, or rinse the outer colored coating off, leaving the hard white shell on the tablets, before swallowing. Following are some recommendations as to brand:

For Women — Centrum, Dr. Art Ulene Nutrition Boost formula for Men & Women, Kroger Complete Extra, OneSource, Rite Aid Whole Source, Safeway Select OmniSource, Spring Valley Advantage, Summit Complete, Twinlab Dualtabs, Walgreens Ultra Choice, YourLife Super Multi-Vitamin.

For Men — Dr. Art Ulene Nutrition Boost Formula for Men & Women, Eckerd Daily Impact Senior, Rite Aid Whole Source Mature Adult, Safeway Select OmniSource Senior, Shaklee Vita-Lea without iron, Twinlab Dualtabs, YourLife Super Multi-Vitamin.

For Older men and women — Dr. Art Ulene Nutrition Boost Formula for Men & Women, Eckerd Daily Impact Senior, Rite Aid Whole Source Mature Adult, Safeway Select OmniSource Senior, Twinlab Dualtabs. (Brand recommendations adapted from the newsletter "Nutrition Action" [see Resources], April 2000 issue.)

3. The third option is to boost the effectiveness of the multi-vitamin/mineral supplement you have chosen. It is often useful to add additional calcium (500 mg), magnesium (250 mg), vitamin C (500 mg), and vitamin E (200 - 400 IU) to the daily tablet described above. These nutrients are usually undersupplied in a multivitamin/mineral supplement, and they are not known to be toxic in these amounts. With the above exceptions in mind, it is a good idea to limit your intake of vitamins and minerals to no more than 150% of the RDA, as large amounts of some vitamins and minerals can be toxic.

Afterword

You now have all the techniques at your disposal to succeed in losing weight or to maintain your present normal weight. The program presented in these pages has worked for a great many of my students, and I am happy to share it with you.

I want to leave you with a thought that has sustained me throughout many years of difficult change and study. According to Yoga, failure is impossible — unless you simply choose not even to try at all. It is the present that matters, and even the tiniest bit of effort is not wasted. If you are trying to change your behavior, your thought patterns, and your view of yourself, it may take some time, but what else could be more exciting? If you concentrate on the present moment, you will never be bored, and you will never fall into the trap of comparing yourself unfavorably with others or with past or future images of yourself. If you continue to practice a little every day, you will grow to love the changes in yourself as your physical and emotional bodies learn to work together to create a healthy, beautiful, happy, and powerful individual.

I wish you the best of success with Yoga and your weight management program.

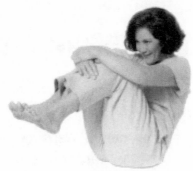

Resources

Nutrition Information / Diet Plans / Calorie Counters / Cookbooks

Nancy Clark's Sports Nutrition Guidebook, 2nd ed., by Nancy Clark (Champaign, IL: Human Kinetics, 1996).

The Nutrition Doctor's A-to-Z Food Counter, by Dr. Ed Blonz (New York: Penguin, 1999).

Prevention Magazine's Nutrition Advisor, by Mark Bricklin (Emmaus, PA: Rodale Press, 1993).

"Nutrition Action" (newsletter of the Center for Science in the Public Interest, 1875 Connecticut Ave, NW, #300, Washington, DC 20009-5729). Up-to-date information for consumers about food safety, nutrition research, healthy eating suggestions, and so on.

Vegetarian Cooking for Everyone, by Deborah Madison (Broadway Books, 1997)

The Complete Vegetarian Cuisine (rev. ed.), by Rose Elliott (Pantheon Books, 1997)

Support Groups and Helpful Websites

Overeaters Anonymous. Consult your local Yellow Pages for referral to a local chapter.

Following are a few helpful Websites available as of the publication of this book. In addition to basic information about healthy weight management, many of these sites offer interactive tools such as individual diet planners and food analysis, a chance to ask experts questions about dieting and nutrition, support chat rooms, and other features. (Because the content of the World Wide Web changes constantly, use search engines to find a current list of helpful sites.)

Cyberdiet.com

Intelihealth.com

Nourishnet.com

Obesity.com

Prevention.com

YourBetterHealth.com

Diet and Weight Loss Professionals

Registered Dieticians

For individualized advice about a weight loss diet, we recommend consulting a registered dietician (RD). These health professionals have fulfilled specific educational requirements, have passed a registration exam, and are a recognized member of the nation's largest organization of nutrition professionals, The American Dietetic Association. Contact them for a referral to a professional in your area.

American Dietetic Association
216 W. Jackson Blvd.
Chicago, IL 60606-6995
Tel: (312) 899-0040 x4750
Fax: (312) 899-4739
Website: www.eatright.org

(800) 366-1655 (toll-free) for recorded messages about current nutrition topics and to get a referral to a registered dietician in your local area.

(900) 225-5267 for individualized answers to your questions from a registered dietician. Charges: $1.95 first minute, $.95 each additional minute, average call four minutes.

Weight Loss Physicians

Call local area hospitals (some have special weight-loss clinics) or look for advertisements in your Yellow Pages or newspaper Health section.

Contact the American Society of Bariatric Physicians. This is a voluntary organization; physicians with the best credentials will also be Diplomates of the American Board of Bariatric Medicine; they will have passed both an on-site, peer-reviewed Patient Care Review and an extensive written and oral board exam.

> **American Society of Bariatric Physicians**
> 5600 S. Quebec St. #109A
> Englewood, CO 80111

(303) 779-4833 to obtain a list of referrals by mail or fax (CO residents in area code 303 call 770-2526, ext. 10); or visit their Website: www.asbp.org

Physician referrals are also available online at www.obesity-news.com

Books on Walking, Swimming, and Cycling

Walking Medicine, by Gary Yanker (McGraw-Hill, 1992)

Walk Aerobics, by Les Snowdon (Overlook Press, 1995)

WALKFIT for a Better Body, by Kathy Smith (Warner Books, 1994)

Fitness Cycling, by Chris Carmichael and Edmund R. Burke (Human Kinetics, 1994)

Power Pacing for Indoor Cycling, by Kristopher Kory and Thomas Seabourne (Human Kinetics, 1999)

Cycling Past 50, by Joe Friel (Human Kinetics, 1998)

All-American Aquatic Handbook, by Jane Katz (Allyn & Bacon, 1996)

Swimming for Total Fitness, by Jane Katz (Main Street Books, rev. ed. 1993)

Complete Book of Swimming, by Dr. Phillip Whitten (Random House, 1994)

Resources from the American Yoga Association

Further information on Yoga is available from the American Yoga Association. To obtain free information about Yoga, including a complete catalog and guidelines for choosing a qualified teacher, visit our website, or send a self-addressed envelope stamped with postage for two ounces to the following address:

American Yoga Association
P.O. Box 19986
Sarasota, FL 34276

If you have a specific question about Yoga and would like a personal reply, write to the address above, or contact us by telephone, fax, or E-mail:

Telephone (941) 927-4977
Fax: (941) 921-9844

E-mail: info@AmericanYogaAssociation.org
Website: AmericanYogaAssociation.org

We offer classes in the Cleveland, Ohio, area. For more information, write or call:

American Yoga Association
P.O. Box 18105
Cleveland Hts, OH 44106
Telephone (216) 556-1313

Books

The American Yoga Association Beginner's Manual (Simon & Schuster, 1987). Complete instructions for over 90 Yoga exercises and breathing techniques; three 10-week curriculum outlines, and chapters on nutrition, philosophy, stress management, nutrition, pregnancy, and more.

The American Yoga Association's New Yoga Challenge (NTC/Contemporary, 1997). Routines for Energy, Strength, Flexibility, Focus, and Stability offer more vigorous Yoga workouts for body and mind. The last chapter, "The Powerful Individual," teaches you how to design your own routine.

The American Yoga Association Wellness Book (Kensington, 1996). A basic routine to maintain health and well-being, plus chapters on how Yoga can specifically help with arthritis, heart disease, back pain, PMS & menopause, weight management, insomnia, headaches, and eight other health conditions.

The American Yoga Association's Yoga for Sports (NTC/Contemporary Books, 2000). A comprehensive book for every athlete, including techniques for bringing the physical and emotional bodies together to attain peak performance. Includes a core routine of exercise, breathing, and meditation, plus specific exercise routines for dozens of individual sports, team sports, and coaches.

Conversations with Swami Lakshmanjoo, Volume I: Aspects of Kashmir Shaivism (American Yoga Association, 1995). Edited transcripts of Alice Christensen's interviews with Swami Lakshmanjoo, talking about his childhood and early years in Yoga, plus some basic concepts in the philosophy of Kashmir Shaivism.

Conversations with Swami Lakshmanjoo, Volume II: The Yamas and Niyamas of Patanjali (American Yoga Association, 1998). Edited transcripts of Alice Christensen's dialogues with Swami Lakshmanjoo about these essential ethical guidelines in Yoga.

Easy Does It Yoga (Fireside/Simon & Schuster, 1999). For those with physical limitations, this book includes instruction in specially adapted Yoga exercises that can be done in a chair or in bed, breathing techniques, and meditation.

The Easy Does It Yoga Trainer's Guide (Kendall-Hunt, 1995). A complete manual for how to begin teaching the Easy Does It Yoga program to adults with physical limitations due to age, convalescence, substance abuse, injury, or obesity. Excellent for health professionals, activities directors, physical therapists, home health aides, and others who work with the elderly or in rehabilitative services.

The Light of Yoga (American Yoga Association, 1997). A chronicle of the unusual circumstances that catapulted Alice Christensen into Yoga practice in the early 1950s, including the teachers and experiences that shaped her first years of study.

Meditation (American Yoga Association, 1994). A collection of excerpts from lectures and classes on the subject of meditation, including a section of questions and answers from students.

20-Minute Yoga Workouts (Ballantine, 1995). Brief routines that anyone can fit into the busiest schedule. Includes chapters on women's issues, toning and shaping, the "20-minute challenge," and workouts to do when you're away from home.

Reflections of Love (American Yoga Association, 1994). A collection of excerpts from Alice Christensen's lectures and classes on the subject of love.

Yoga of the Heart: Ten Ethical Principles for Gaining Limitless Growth, Confidence, and Achievement (Daybreak/Rodale Books, 1998). A clear, direct presentation of ten essential ethics — Nonviolence, Truthfulness, Nonstealing, Celibacy, Nonhoarding, Purity, Contentment, Tolerance, Study, and Remembrance — that help a person realize the power and support of joining the physical and spiritual bodies. Each chapter includes suggestions for how to start practicing, common pitfalls along the way, and many examples from students' experiences and mythology to illustrate the journey.

Audiotapes

Complete Relaxation and Meditation with Alice Christensen. A two-tape audiocassette program that features three guided meditation sessions of varying lengths, including instruction in a seated posture, plus a discussion of meditation experiences.

The "I Love You" Meditation Technique. This technique begins with the experience of a more conscious connection with the breath through love. It then extends this feeling throughout the body and mind in relaxation and meditation. This tape teaches you the beauty of loving yourself and it removes unseen fear.

Videotapes

Basic Yoga. A complete introduction to Yoga that includes exercise, breathing, and relaxation and meditation techniques. Provides detailed instruction in all the techniques including variations for more or less flexibility, plus a special limbering routine and back-strengthening exercises. Features a 30-minute daily routine demonstrated in the setting of a Yoga class.

Conversations with Swami Lakshmanjoo. A set of three videotapes in which Alice Christensen introduces Swami Lakshmanjoo and talks with him about his background, the philosophy of Kashmir Shaivism, and other topics in Yoga. (Some material corresponds to Volume I of the book *Aspects of Kashmir Shaivism* described above.)

The Yamas and Niyamas: A Videotape Study Program. A complete set of 25 videotapes of Alice Christensen's comprehensive lectures on the ethical guidelines that form the cornerstone of Yoga philosophy and practice.

The Hero in Yoga: A Videotape Study Program. A series of 24 videotaped lectures by Alice Christensen on Joseph Campbell's landmark text *The Hero With a Thousand Faces,* showing how the adventure of the hero, represented in mythologies all over the globe, parallels the Yoga student's search for self-actualization.

How to Choose a Qualified Yoga Teacher

So far, no national or international certification program for yoga teachers exists, and it is unlikely that it will, because of the traditional nature of Yoga instruction. For many thousands of years, Yoga was transmitted from teacher to student on a one-to-one basis; only comparatively recently has Yoga been offered in a group class format. Advanced practice of Yoga still is best undertaken on a one-to-one basis, if you are lucky enough to find a competent teacher who is willing to teach you. In my opinion, teaching Yoga should not be viewed as a hobby or a sideline undertaken by someone who reads a couple of books and decides to become a Yoga teacher; he or she must be under the constant supervision of his or her personal Yoga teacher. This relationship between teacher and student is taken very seriously by both parties and is never entered into lightly.

People are constantly asking us to recommend teachers in their area. Because of my belief in the strict training required for the teaching of Yoga, I have made it a policy never to recommend a teacher unless I have trained the person. I cannot take responsibility for other people's teaching. This does not mean that there are no competent teachers available; you may just have to search a little harder. If you are not sure where to start looking, inquire about adult education programs at local schools; look for flyers posted in local health food stores and bookstores or notices in community papers; and inquire at dance and massage studios.

In the following paragraphs, I have outlined what I believe are the minimum requirements for a competent teacher of Yoga.

1. Daily practice of Yoga exercise, breathing, and meditation. No one can make progress in Yoga without a serious commitment to daily practice. A teacher must have this support in order to build the solid foundation of experience that is required before he or she can show others how to achieve that experience; daily practice is also needed to maintain the strength and health necessary for the extra demands of teaching.

2. Regular contact with a teacher. No teacher can work effectively in a vacuum, and no one becomes so advanced that he or she does not need the guidance and support of his or her own teacher.

3. Study of the important Yoga texts. Study is one of the five observances that are part of the essential eight "limbs" of Yoga practice (see #4, below). A teacher needs to have an intensive background of study that includes Patanjali's *Yoga Sutras*, the *Hatha Yoga Pradipika*, the *Bhagavad Gita*, and all world philosophies, at the very least.

4. Ethical behavior. The five *yamas* (meaning "restraints": nonviolence, truthfulness, nonstealing, periods of celibacy, nonhoarding) and the five *niyamas* (meaning "observances": purity, contentment, tolerance, study, remembrance) are the first two limbs in Patanjali's system of classical Yoga (called "Ashtanga Yoga"). The remaining six limbs are 1) physical exercises *(asana)*, 2) breathing techniques *(pranayama)*, 3) withdrawal of the mind from the senses *(pratyahara)*, 4) concentration, defined as selective and voluntary dishabituation *(dharana)*, 5) meditation *(dhyana)*, and 6) absorption, or ultimate union with the self *(samadhi)*. My teacher Lakshmanjoo once said that, like a child developing in the womb whose limbs grow all at once, rather than one by one, these eight limbs must be developed simultaneously.

The ethical guidelines of the yamas and niyamas are a part of Yoga practice not for moralistic reasons but because they support and protect the student during the unfolding of personal experience in meditation. A teacher needs this support and protection for the same reasons as well as to help reduce the interference of personal ego in the teaching process.

An ethical Yoga teacher conducts classes in a responsible, safe, and aware manner; organizes classes that are not too large for each student to receive individual attention; and never pushes students beyond their limitations. Sexual involvement with students is absolutely prohibited.

5. A healthy vegetarian diet. Although you do not need to be a vegetarian to practice Yoga, a Yoga teacher must conform to different standards. Someone who is taking responsibility for teaching others how to use Yoga meditation techniques must have the steadiness and nonviolent attitude that can only be attained through a vegetarian diet. It goes without saying that a teacher should not smoke or use drugs (other than prescription medication) or misuse alcohol.

6. Training in basic anatomy and the effects of Yoga techniques. A teacher must be able to vary the techniques according to each student's ability and know how to advise students with common medical conditions such as hypertension, arthritis, and back problems. I also believe that a teacher should be able to recognize when a student needs professional psychological counseling and be familiar with community services to which to refer the student.

7. Ability to separate Yoga from religion. I have seen many poor-quality instructors take on the trappings and robes of Hinduism or some other religion to give themselves an authority through packaging rather than through the authenticity of their own Yoga practice. This practice severely misrepresents Yoga. Yoga is not a religion; it predates Hinduism — as well as all known religious practices — and its techniques have been used throughout the world. Yoga is a system of nonreligious, transcultural techniques that can develop greater self-knowledge and awareness. Unlike a religion, Yoga does not require adherence to certain creeds or beliefs, nor does it require obeisance to any particular prophet or god. Yoga is not ritualistic, nor is it occult. The texts of Yoga are not scriptures but rather handbooks or guidelines of how to use the techniques safely and what kinds of experiences might be possible. Everyone has a right to their personal religious beliefs, but a teacher must never impose his or her personal beliefs on students in a Yoga class.

About the American Yoga Association

The American Yoga Association teaches a comprehensive and balanced program of Yoga that includes the Hatha Yoga exercises and breathing techniques as well as meditation. Rather than stressing physical culture for its own sake, our core curriculum acknowledges the deeper possibilities of Yoga by teaching meditation and by encouraging the inner-directed awareness that eventually leads to greater self-knowledge. This reliance on individual experience and feeling is a central theme in the science of Yoga, and it underlies the philosophical system of Kashmir Shaivism which supports our line of teaching. Our goal is to offer the highest quality Yoga instruction possible. There are two American Yoga Association Centers in the United States.

About the Author

Alice Christensen stands out as a Yoga teacher with the rare ability to make the often-complex ideas and techniques of Yoga accessible to our Western outlook and lifestyle. She established the American Yoga Association in 1968, the first nonprofit organization in the United States dedicated to education in Yoga.

She has consistently presented Yoga in a clear, classical manner for over forty years. She presents Yoga without dogma or prescription, as a potent avenue for individual inquiry. She has designed programs of Yoga that can be used to enhance any lifestyle. Whether the goal is to maintain health or to explore the nature of the self, her programs can be used to achieve a wide range of goals.

Index